ANTHROPOLOGY OF NURSING

This book aims to introduce nurses and other healthcare professionals to how anthropology can help them understand nursing as a profession and as a culture.

Drawing on key anthropological concepts, the book facilitates the understanding and critical consideration of nursing practice, as seen across a wide range of health care contexts, and which impacts the delivery of appropriate care for service users. Considering the fields in which nurses work, the book argues that in order for nurses to optimise their roles as deliverers of patient care, they must not only engage with the realities of the cultural world of the patient, but also that of their own multi-professional cultural environment.

The only book currently in the field on anthropology of nursing, this book will be a valuable resource for nursing students at all academic levels, especially where they can pursue specific modules in the subject, as well as those other students pursuing medical anthropology courses. As well as this, it will be an essential text for those post-graduate students who wish to consider alternative world views from anthropology and their application in nursing and healthcare, in addition to their undertaking ethnographic research to explore nursing in all its fields of practice.

Karen Holland is Editor in Chief of the journal *Nurse Education in Practice* and holds a position as part-time lecturer at the University of Salford in the School of Health and Society. She has written and edited a number of books for nurses and other health professionals.

ANTHROPOLOGY OF NURSING

Exploring Cultural Concepts in Practice

Edited by Karen Holland

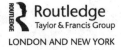

Routledge
Taylor & Francis Group

LONDON AND NEW YORK

First published 2020
by Routledge
2 Park Square, Milton Park, Abingdon, Oxon OX14 4RN

and by Routledge
52 Vanderbilt Avenue, New York, NY 10017

Routledge is an imprint of the Taylor & Francis Group, an informa business

British Library Cataloguing in Publication Data
A catalogue record for this book is available from the British Library

Library of Congress Cataloging-in-Publication Data
A catalog record has been requested for this book

ISBN: 978-1-138-91279-3 (hbk)
ISBN: 978-1-138-91280-9 (pbk)
ISBN: 978-1-315-69178-7 (ebk)

Typeset in Bembo
by Taylor & Francis Books

This book is dedicated to the late Emeritus Professor of Medical Sociology, Joel Richman, to whom I owe a huge debt of gratitude for opening my eyes to other possibilities of being a nurse and how nursing could be seen. His support as I began to explore the nursing world from a unique perspective of culture, rituals and ethnography was immense, and he was an incredible knowledgeable supervisor. This book therefore is steeped in my experience of learning with him and also exploring my own 'anthropological lens' to nursing.

CONTENTS

List of boxes   *ix*
List of contributors   *x*
Acknowledgements   *xi*
Preface   *xiii*

1 Principles of anthropology for nursing and health care   1
   Karen Holland

2 Culture and nursing: an anthropological perspective   20
   Karen Holland

3 Researching culture: principles of ethnography and ethnographic
   fieldwork   36
   Karen Holland

4 Time and space in the context of nursing work   51
   Karen Holland

5 Rituals, rites and nursing practice   68
   Karen Holland

6 Transition and initiation: the student nurse   81
   Karen Holland

7 Nursing work within nursing culture: images and reality   99
   Karen Holland

8 Dirt, pollution and the body: meaning for nursing practice   113
   Karen Holland

9 Withdrawal of treatment in the critical care unit: insights into a trajectory of dying and death 129
Jenni Templeman

10 Nursing and culture: language, knowledge and power 145
Benny Goodman

Index 162

BOXES

6.1 Aspects of an initiation (as defined by La Fontaine 1985)   91
6.2 Examples of bounded placement experiences for student nurses   91

CONTRIBUTORS

Benny Goodman is an independent scholar, formerly a lecturer with the School of Nursing and Midwifery at the University of Plymouth. He has written and co-written a number of articles and text books focusing on the social sciences and sustainability in health.

Karen Holland is Editor in Chief of the journal *Nurse Education in Practice* and holds a position as part-time lecturer at the University of Salford in the School of Health and Society. She has written and edited a number of books for nurses and other health professionals.

Jenni Templeman is a senior lecturer and programme lead in the Faculty of Health and Social Care at the University of Chester. Jenni has written chapters for several books and is research active.

ACKNOWLEDGEMENTS

There are many people I have acknowledged and thanked in the introduction to the book, and all have made a contribution to my journey to this point in time. However there are specific 'others' that I have to acknowledge as contributing to my ongoing learning and engagement with the subject of this book.

One is the late Dr Sue Philpin whose work on rituals in nursing and ethnographic research in a nursing ITU, remains an incredible addition to the literature bridging nursing and anthropology. To have a conversation with her, or reading her work, without needing a dictionary of anthropological concepts and language was a joy. She travelled on a parallel journey and has been very much missed. Her work however still continues to have an impact on my thinking.

I have to thank Professor Emeritus Tony Warne for his ongoing support and friendship over the years, including his invaluable engagement with my interest in anthropology and nursing as a post-graduate supervisor, as well as his support in numerous roles and research projects. His own doctorate study and later work offered an insight into the context of nursing and health care within the broader culture of the health care organizations.

Professor Emeritus Martin Johnson provided me with an opportunity to be challenged on some of my thinking around ethnography, as I co-supervised with him those doctorate students who chose this methodology for their research. His extensive knowledge of nursing history and understanding of nursing as situated in his own doctorate study has also been invaluable.

I wish to acknowledge all the undergraduate students that have taken part in my research studies and teaching over time and to those engaged in informal dialogue about their experiences whilst 'in the field' and as key informants into their world. These 'realist tales', have enabled me to gain an understanding of how their experiences of an overall nursing culture and the subcultures they experienced during their varied clinical placements supported their journey to becoming a registered and qualified nurse.

I also wish to thank those post-graduate students I have supervised who have followed an ethnography journey to successful completion of the doctorate studies. This enabled me to re-read those amazing ethnographies of experts in the field talked about in this book, as well as gaining new insights into fieldwork experiences in different nursing contexts.

I wish to acknowledge the trust that the team at Routledge placed in me to deliver this book, and their support when things did not go to plan as it were. I was privileged to have them publish my *Cultural Awareness in Nursing and Health Care* book and knew that given their incredible portfolio of anthropology-related books there was nowhere else I would have chosen to publish this book.

Especial thanks go to the Routledge team:

Grace McInnes, Carolina Atunes and Ruth Anderson for their amazing support during the whole journey.

Thanks go to Katie Golsby for copy-editing my work.

Veronica Richards for the design of the book including the beautiful cover which many will recognise if you have ever visited Angkor Wat.

Last but never least is my ongoing thanks to my husband Terry who has not only lived with me and my passion for nursing education and learning about cultures and anthropology for 44 years, but also for sharing in my travel experiences to visit some of the most amazing countries worldwide and meeting so many wonderful peoples that live there. We are of course planning more!

PREFACE

The introduction to this book is very much about how it came to be written and how I, in my place as it were as both an insider and outsider in relation to the culture of nursing, came to the decision of viewing it with an anthropological lens. It is a personal narrative underpinned by an insight into people and experiences that have shaped my knowledge and interest in culture and anthropology. I like to think of them as 'snapshots' in time.

I need to state from the outset that I am not an anthropologist in the tradition of the eminent Malinowski and other major ethnographers. Some would also say that I am not even a nurse anthropologist. However what I do have is experience of undertaking ethnographic research in the fields of nursing practice and education as well as many years of supporting student and qualified nurses to engage in learning in these two fields. This insider experience of being a nurse myself and being 'of the nursing culture', has been invaluable in the development of the proposal for this book, as well as the writing of it.

I have had a life-long interest in learning about other cultures of the world, which began at the age of six years when my uncle introduced me to the world of the National Geographic magazine! It was only much later in my life that I was very fortunate to be able to visit some of these wonderful countries and meet some amazing people and cultures, but not unfortunately in the tradition of Margaret Mead and others. However because of how these visits took place I was fortunate to be able to engage with people away from the 'tourist' pathways, and learnt that regardless of what culture one belongs to, as a woman I was able to communicate with other women who spoke only their own language and dialects, about their life and their families.

I first became interested in the potential of nursing as a culture when undertaking a part-time nursing degree at, what was then known as, Manchester Polytechnic in 1987. The course was an incredible journey and involved amazing learning opportunities, including being introduced to medical sociology and anthropology as well as ethnography as both research and writing. Access to learning about major ethnographies such as those of Branislaw Malinowski (*Argonauts of the Western Pacific*), Evans-Pritchard (*The Nuer*) and Margaret Mead (*Coming of Age in Samoa*) together with the more popular readings and wonderful tales of

Nigel Barley and his ethnographic fieldwork experiences among the Dowayo people in Northern Cameroon, stimulated my long-standing interest in different cultures of the world.

During my graduate studies we had to complete an actual research project and I knew it had to be an ethnography of some kind. During my reading about nursing and sociology I came across the most thought-provoking paper by Chapman (1983) called 'Ritual and Rational Action in Hospitals' and knew as soon as I had read it that here was a fascinating concept to consider in relation to nursing. My research supervisor was the late Emeritus Professor of Medical Sociology, Professor Joel Richman, himself an ethnographer of street administration, i.e. Traffic Wardens, who encouraged my interest and supported the proposal – the outcome was for me the most wonderful experience of 'doing research in the field' at a time when nursing and ethnographic research were new to each other, and most certainly in determining whether ritual and nursing had something to offer each other. As a result of that early work and with the wonderful support of the editor at that time it was published in the *Journal of Advanced Nursing* in 1993 under the wonderful title of: 'An ethnographic study of nursing culture as an exploration for determining the existence of a system of ritual'. During this time I became involved in teaching sociology and some basic aspects of anthropology to Project 2000 students; the curriculum at the time giving us wonderful opportunities to expand our minds and thinking as well as that of the students. I subsequently undertook a course gaining my teaching qualification, led by a Programme Director who was a sociologist and enabled me to maintain my ongoing interest in the boundaries between sociology and anthropology whilst looking through a new lens of teaching and learning as well as analysing the curriculum as a cultural artefact. As a result of needing to continue studying as part of my work role, I persuaded the School management team to support my post-graduate studies in Medical Social Anthropology at Keele University. There followed two of the most special years of my career, in expanding what I already knew to a new place in anthropological knowledge. Our course tutors were incredibly knowledgeable and experienced in their various fields, such as Dr Ursula Sharma (now Professor), Dr Alan Prout (now Professor Emeritus) and the wonderful late Professor Emeritus Ronald (Ronnie) Frankenberg who taught the same course at Brunel University London. I recall a particularly challenging brief he gave us, to present our views (underpinned by anthropological evidence) on the concepts of Naked and Nude – my midwifery colleague and I certainly brought to the session not only our professional experiences with women but also our personal perspective as women! This challenging of students to bring anthropological research and historical ethnographies to underpin our discussions in relation to our professional realities was such a wonderful experience.

My interest, by the time I started to think of undertaking this MSc course, had expanded to look at nursing from many different perspectives, and as a lecturer and personal tutor to student nurses I had begun to consider that there was more to their journey to becoming a qualified nurse than simply passing exams or gaining clinical practice experience. This became my next big project, and although my tutors were not always sure that my understanding of rites of passage or transition rites could be related to ritual as in anthropology, I received much support from my supervisors to look at the possible relationship. I gained my MSc in Medical Social Anthropology and have always been grateful for the collegial relationship we had as students with our course tutors, as they were often heard to say that we brought experience of the 'real world' into the classroom to share with each other and in turn themselves. My research dissertation was eventually turned into a new publication on student nurse transition (Holland 1999) which was for me another major step forward for raising awareness of ethnography as well as anthropology.

I had already continued my interest in cultural issues, especially those that impacted on the way nursing and health care were delivered in practice, and designed and then taught a new Transcultural Nursing Module in a degree course for qualified nurses. I came to realise that there were no textbooks that were specific to our health care context in the UK so a colleague and I developed a proposal based on our collective teaching notes and wide reading and it was accepted for a new book in the field of cultural awareness for nursing and healthcare. By the time it was published I knew I wanted to know more about nursing as a culture, and although there were some like-minded colleagues who communicated with me about this, there did not seem to be any major drive towards learning from anthropology to understand nursing. The life-saving edited book by Holden & Littlewood (1991), *Anthropology and Nursing*, had already made a substantial addition to our teaching and was a clear signpost that it was possible for evidence that supported an anthropology of nursing to be added to through further research. The book offered a number of chapters by different authors, exploring aspects of nursing culture and anthropology in different countries and contexts; although Littlewood had also offered nursing a model based on 'the incorporation of medical anthropology into the nursing process' (Littlewood 1989).

I continued to teach and broaden my knowledge and understanding of cultural issues and published a second edition of the *Cultural Awareness in Nursing and Health Care* book (Holland & Hogg 2010) but my career and family life took me on new pathways. Following four years of part-time doctorate studies, exploring the world of the student nurse and nursing work, I unfortunately had to make a major life-changing decision to halt my studies, due to the major pressure of having a parent with cancer who needed more of my time until her death, as well as my two growing children and a husband plus by then a full-time job and a new senior role at work and as a journal editor. It was the hardest decision I have had to make but I resolved then and there to continue my interest and teaching in anthropology and nursing culture, and possibly return at some future date to recommence studying. This did happen much later than I had envisaged and also not through undertaking further post-graduate studies.

Not wanting to lose all my experience and learning, through my research studies, supervision of post-graduate students with an interest in ethnography, culture and anthropology and other interests, as well as a wide range of skills I had now acquired in writing books and editing a journal, I decided to develop a proposal for this book which was after external review accepted for taking forward by the publisher.

I had also successfully completed a third revision of *Cultural Awareness in Nursing and Health Care*, an endeavour which I had started with a colleague with similar interests and published first in 2001, and then again with a second edition in 2010 which to our amazement was also translated into Japanese. The latest third edition (Holland 2017), however, I had to sadly manage on my own as my good friend and colleague, as well as co-author, Dr Christine Hogg died five years ago (6 January 2014) at the age of 53.

Although this narrative is a shortened one, I hope that the reader can see that my journey through learning and knowledge, including periods of 'being in the field', has been embedded in aspects of social and cultural anthropology, and this will be translated through the chapters of this book which I hope will introduce others to an enhanced understanding of its value to our understanding about nursing as both profession and work.

I have gathered evidence to support the way in which we can learn from modern ethnographic studies and established ethnographies, as well as engaging in some discussion about the evidence itself. I have also attempted to define what **'nursing anthropology'** could be as a field of study, and offer two possible definitions which I hope will be a trigger for readers to explore for themselves the possibilities for establishing such a field. I wish to stress that the book is based on my interpretation of significant events that have taken place in nursing history based on anthropological principles, as well as literature that I have researched and discovered, and then 'pulled together' as it were to establish an introduction to anthropology as it relates to nursing in all its fields of practice.

It is the kind of book that I would have liked early in my research journey, one that gives direction to possibilities and alternative ways of viewing nursing as well as providing an accumulation of different kinds of evidence to begin a journey through nursing using an 'anthropological lens'. It is most certainly not a definitive text, as there is much more that I have discovered from which we can learn and explore in relation to nursing as both profession and work.

This book is therefore for those undergraduates who may have specific modules in the subject, and especially for those post graduates and faculty members who look for alternative views and 'lenses' with which to study nursing as a field of practice or to support their actual practice as a nurse in the various fields in which they work. It is an exploration and it is a beginning.

Structure of the book

In order to begin this journey the book has been structured to enable the major principles and theoretical concepts related to anthropology to be explored first, followed by chapters focusing on more specific aspects of nursing and anthropological concepts. There are in addition two invited author chapters where the content and context offer a different anthropological lens on the world of nursing and nursing work. I am very grateful for their invaluable contribution.

References

Chapman G E (1983) Ritual and rational action in hospitals, *Journal of Advanced Nursing*, 8, 13–20.

Holden P & LittlewoodJ (1991) *Anthropology and Nursing*, Routledge, London.

Holland K (1999) A journey to becoming: The student nurse in transition, *Journal of Advanced Nursing*, 29(1), 1461–1470.

Holland K (2017) *Cultural Awareness in Nursing and Health Care. An Introductory Text*, 3rd Edition, Routledge, London.

Holland K & HoggC (2010) *Cultural Awareness in Nursing and Health Care: An Introductory Text*, 2nd Edition, Routledge, London.

Littlewood J (1989) A model for nursing using anthropological literature, *International Journal of Nursing Studies*, 26(3), 221–229.

1

PRINCIPLES OF ANTHROPOLOGY FOR NURSING AND HEALTH CARE

Karen Holland

Introduction

This chapter establishes an understanding of anthropology as a discipline with its own body of knowledge that can enable us to utilise it as a lens to study nursing and health care. The key concepts that anthropologists have used to explain their understanding of how people live in various societies will be explored and it will set the scene for the other chapters which draw on these concepts to explore nursing in more depth. It is noted that we need to look at both anthropology *for* nursing (how anthropological concepts can help us in understanding the work that nurses undertake) and also the anthropology *of* nursing, where the focus is on nursing as a culture in itself which can contribute to the anthropological literature. They are in fact intertwined, as culture is itself a major anthropological concept. These differences will become clearer as the chapters unfold.

Principles of anthropology

What do we mean when we talk about anthropology? There has been much debate since anthropology came into its own as a recognised discipline as to what knowledge can be considered 'anthropological'. Lavenda & Schultz (2010, p. 3) note that historically anthropology '*has been divided into four major subfields: biological anthropology, cultural anthropology, linguistic anthropology and archaeology*'. The main focus in this book is on cultural anthropology or as many define it: social and cultural anthropology (Monaghan & Just 2000; Eriksen 2015). Others such as Bueno (2012) and Lavenda & Schultz (2010) point out that these two actually relate to the two main countries where anthropology developed, namely cultural in the USA and social in Great Britain. There is also a close link to studies about cultures in the discipline of sociology (Bueno 2012), and in some of the chapters such as that on ritual and transition (Chapter 5), there is clearly an enhanced understanding of various aspects of nursing as a culture through an exploration of both disciplines.

We will, however, touch upon knowledge from one or two of the other anthropology subfields, in particular to what has become known as a major area of study in relation to health care, that is medical anthropology. This field of study focuses on factors related to health and illness or as Pool & Geissler (2005) state: '*Medical anthropology describes, interprets and critically appraises the relationships between culture, behaviour, health and disease, and places health and illness in the broader context of cultural, social, political, economic and historical processes*' (p. 29). Given that medicine and nursing co-exist in similar contexts, there will be examples where this causes dissonance, such as in the care of the patient and also the wider setting of their professional domains.

As the book focuses on social and cultural anthropology, we need to establish what are the core areas of the discipline to focus on as they relate to nursing, as it is an impossible undertaking to discuss all the issues and debates pertaining to such a vast topic. It has already been stated in the Preface that the key areas will focus on nursing as care and nursing as work, both of which have their own areas of literature and critical debate.

The first and major concept to consider is that of Culture, which again has a number of aspects related to nursing (see Chapter 2), whilst others such as ritual, time, space, organisation of society and work, beliefs and values arise from how culture is viewed both inside and outside of its boundaries. The second major concept is how cultures were and are studied: ethnographies or ethnographic research. This is the focus of Chapter 3.

Culture and anthropology

Because of the various ways in which culture is now considered, it is important that we begin by examining one of the most established definitions of culture, which remains influential in determining how nursing has been considered in various research studies. The definition that influenced much of our early understanding of the work of anthropologists is that by E. B. Tylor in 1871, namely that culture is: '*That complex whole which includes knowledge, beliefs, art, law, morals, custom, and any other capabilities and habits acquired by man as a member of society.*' We take it to mean that the use of the word 'man' in his definition takes into account both genders, where 'man' refers to a human being. This can of course be much debated. The main issue to take from this definition is that he saw culture as 'a complex whole', incorporating those aspects he defined, which would in fact remain the main definition for some years.

If we re-examine this definition from a woman's point of view, which clearly reflected the period in history when men were the dominant sex in any discourse concerning art and science, then it could be argued that in any cultural 'ethnography' or report of the time that it was predominantly the male viewpoint that was explored and considered and not female. Women were also constrained by the wider society in which they lived, and were not at the time noted for their ethnographies.

However, we know, before 1871, that women were already making their voices heard in society, especially about nursing and care of the sick. Women such as Elizabeth Fry, Mrs Bedford Fenwick and Florence Nightingale each had their own agenda with regards to caring for the sick and training those who would care for them. Their work was set against the religious debates of the period in the middle 1800s, as well as the suffragette movement and the attempt to gain a vote for women. Bullough & Bullough (1964) writing about *The Emergence of Modern Nursing*, stated that by '*the 1870's the foundation of modern nursing had been laid and with it the foundation of the modern hospital*' (p. 112).

We can only gain an insight into the culture in which nurses worked and nursing developed during this period in history from the words that were left by those who were educated and able to access resources with which to get their writing published; women such as Florence Nightingale. She left many pamphlets or small books such as Notes on Nursing and Notes on Hospitals in 1859.

Others also wrote their accounts of life as they saw it; an interesting one called *Eastern Hospitals and English Nurses*, by A Lady Volunteer, states it is a narrative of 12 months' experience in the hospitals of Koulali and Scutari (A Lady Volunteer 1856 – who was later found to be a lady called Frances Margaret Taylor: see https://archive.org/details/easternhosp itals00unse and below). Her insights into this developing 'nursing world', through her observations and her experiences of literally 'being in field', bring to life the conditions at that time. Although not what we would now assign the title 'an ethnography', it raises the question: 'does this work?' and others like it meet the definition of ethnography as the 'written product', based on the result of fieldwork as defined by Van Maanen (1988). In other words – does it describe the culture (nursing), the people (nurses and others) and context (hospitals and war zones) so that those reading it can see this? Although of course Taylor at the time did not see herself as this 'ethnographic fieldworker' but sought to raise awareness in the public of the need for 'a proper system of female nursing' (Preface to her 1856 version) through her narrative. We will return to this debate of whether some of these early publications demonstrate qualities of an ethnography in Chapter 3.

Reading the publisher information about this unknown lady it appears that she was in fact one of Florence Nightingale's earliest nursing recruits:

> The author of this remarkable pseudonymous two-volume, eyewitness account of Florence Nightingale's nursing in the Crimean War was really Frances Margaret Taylor. She was the daughter of an Anglican vicar, who served the poor in his Lincolnshire parish. In 1854 Taylor was one of the earliest nurses to be recruited by Nightingale, and her book is an account of the work she and her fellow nurses carried out for the war-wounded in the hospitals at Scutari and Koulali. She describes the original filthy conditions at the old Turkish hospital, and the problems that the Lady with the Lamp and her nurses had to overcome. (Naval Military Press 2009)

Women such as Florence Nightingale had also taken an interest in what was happening in other societies, in particular, as Hagey (1988) described in her presentation of a paper entitled 'Note on the aboriginal races of Australia' that she gave at 'the annual meeting of the National Association for the Promotion of Social Science, held at York' (p. 1). Her paper, however, on reading it (Nightingale 1865: accessed at https://archive.org/details/nightingale) was in fact more akin to a narrative analysis of ongoing reports/documents from a Roman Catholic Bishop Salvadore who she communicated with as she sought to understand the impact possible training has on the improved health of Australian Aborigines. Her paper offers quote after quote (like a 'tell it as it is' narrative) from his report to her on all manner of his insights and experiences related to Australian Aborigines at that time in history, and her conclusion on the benefit of European civilisation on their lives and culture is a negative one as she agrees with Bishop Salvado in this statement which I include in so far as it illustrates the background to a cultural situation that has not been shared previously, was of its time in history and in fact still has lessons for today's society when discussing integration and assimilation of culture and cultural norms of the more dominant population – as well as offering an insight into the colonial perception and views of race dominant at that time in British history which also impacted on the work of early anthropologists:

> Upon the Australian races European civilisation (Christian in name, but far from Christian in reality) has come suddenly and with overwhelming force. It has found them utterly unable to hold their own against it, equally incapable of joining with and flowing onward with the advancing tide; and therefore these races have been, since the contact first took place, and still are, going down before and beneath its, to them, destructive progress. If their condition had been less degraded, or if the tone of our civilisation had been less overbearing, self-seeking, and oppressive, or even if the irruption of the one upon the other had been less sudden and less violent, the result might have been different. But it is vain to speculate upon what might have been; we know, too well unhappily, what has been taking place, steadily and surely, from the moment when Europeans first set foot upon the Australian continent until this present time. The native races sink down and perish at our presence. (Nightingale 1865)

This observation could be viewed as quite radical in its day, but Florence Nightingale was not one for holding back expressing her views or sharing others', when it came to impact of how people lived, or how governments impacted on the health of nations. She wrote many publications and presented some of this forward thinking to the National Association for the Promotion of Social Science which, according to Huch (1985), during its time (1857–1886) made various important contributions to Victorian Health Reform. It must be remembered, however, that much of her early work was set against the Colonial period where Australia was a British colony and under British rule, so like many other similar countries in the same situation, there was the drive to 'civilise' Aboriginal people through 'conversion to Christian beliefs' and when Nightingale-trained nurses arrived in Australia there was *'no thought of training Aboriginal nurses'* (Best & Fredericks 2014, p. 59).

This example of Florence Nightingale's perspective on another culture and community offers us an insight into how social science was being recognised in Victorian times and also, from members' writings, an insight into the culture of that period as it related to health. Florence Nightingale was, it could be argued, an 'armchair' anthropologist, who wrote and analysed documents about other cultures and their way of life, and made assumptions based on these from her perspective.

A paper by Sera-Shriar (2014) offers an excellent insight into this role which he identifies was part of the early development of anthropology in Britain in the 19th century and which then led to the later *'professional ethnographer and fieldworker'* (p. 28). He stresses that the role of an armchair anthropologist who relied on external data and no fieldwork, was not *'a passive pursuit, with minimal analytical reflection that simply synthesized the materials of other writers.'* He also stresses that: *'Practitioners in the 19th century were highly attuned to the problems associated with their research techniques and continually sought to transform their methodologies* (p. 26)'.

I am not making a claim here that Florence Nightingale deliberately set out to be an 'armchair anthropologist' but given what we can see from her writings and the interpretations of others of this work – such as Gourley (2004) in relation to India – it is evident that through her eyes we can now see in Geertz' (1973) terms, 'slices of culture' or 'thick descriptions' of parts of a culture, and these focus on health and sanitation and education, especially of women. I will return to further discussion of these terms in Chapter 3.

An interesting foreword by Vogel (1989) in the renewed publication of Ruth Benedict's *The Chrysanthemum and the Sword: Patterns of Japanese Culture* noted that Benedict (1946) at the time she started her study could not access the field of Japanese culture, because the USA was at war with Japan (1944). The impact this had on her work and other social scientists of the time, was to undertake to '*study culture from a distance*' (Vogel 1989, p. ix), and she contends that the '*method was not so different from what any historian ordinarily does; to make the most creative imaginative use possible of written documents.*'

Now I do not choose to have a debate here on the difference between an historical account or desk top research, but given that Benedict's written book became famous for its insight into Japanese culture for some years, yet she did not set foot in the country, I see a parallel with the writing of Nightingale about a number of health issues in different countries like Australia, India and Africa. Nightingale's writings based on information shared by both English and Indian colleagues for example offer an incredible insight into what life was like regarding many health, social and political issues set against the backdrop of India at the time without having set foot in the country. Regardless of this Gourley (2004) in her analysis of Nightingale's work and the description of life in India has presented an amazing insight into this period of time in history, in her book: *Florence Nightingale and the Health of the Raj*.

There was, however, one major difference in relation to Benedict's work, as Vogel states: she actually undertook some interviewing of Japanese immigrants to America (already living there pre-war) to gain an added insight into some of the issues she found from her searching and analysis of written documents. However, she was criticised later about her findings about aspects of Japanese life and culture, by those social scientists who had undertaken actual fieldwork in Japan (Vogel 1989), as they did not feel she actually offered a 'realistic' picture of the Japanese people. The main point here is the similarity in offering us an insight into 'cultural scenes' from other countries, to Florence Nightingale and her nurses' legacy, with written narratives, without actually stepping foot as it were in that country.

Documentary analysis, as we will see in Chapter 3, has become an important aspect of studying culture, with documents being considered as 'cultural artefacts' or, as Hodder (1998) refers to them, as being part of a 'material culture' (p. 114).

We can see from evidence that Florence Nightingale's correspondence concerning important health issues was in the main with men, of various nationalities, who valued her insight and correspondence. She later of course wrote what has become a body of evidence on the health issues of the period, including her papers on the nature of nursing and the structured approach to the education and training for nurses for the profession. You could argue that she has become part of the 'folklore' that is part of the cultural history of nursing.

Hagey (1988) believes that Nightingale's '*understanding of culture was the same as what was available and in circulation in those times*', in particular related to race and where people were in terms of their evolution in relation to other societies. Hagey (1988, p. 3) cites the work of Stocking (1968) in relation to culture, in that it was, before 1900, '*associated with the progressive accumulation of the characteristic manifestations of human creativity: art, science, knowledge, refinement – those things that freed man from control by nature, by environment, by reflex, by instinct, by habit or by custom*'.

For the purpose of this book we are focusing our interpretation of culture on the wider anthropological definitions than that relating to Tylor's early definition. F W Voget (2009) stated that the early definitions of culture were very much linked to evolutionists' view of man, and that early anthropologists linked their understanding to social behaviour and in turn psychology. It was only later that the discipline created 'new linkages with sociology' and the 'rise of social interactionism' (p. 943).

The shift from seeing a person on their own, outwith the society in which they lived, led Franz Boas (1962) for example to state that '*We cannot treat the individual as an isolated unit. He must be studied in his social setting*' and he was very insistent that it was only by doing this that one could see '*whether any generally valid laws exist that govern the life of society*' (p. 15).

The ongoing debates on the meaning of culture led to what became known as 'functionalism' or a functionalist view of culture, in particular as Voget (2009) states that interpreted by Malinowski (1954) and Radcliffe-Brown (1935) in their studies. His definition of this viewpoint is that '*cultures were structured systems and their basic processes were largely maintenance operations … the basic processes of culture were not historic, but processes of internal and reciprocating connections …*'. He states that functionalism became divided into two 'streams' – with Malinowski stressing the relation between common biological needs and culture, whilst Radcliffe-Brown emphasised the structured interconnections and maintenance processes of the social system (p. 950).

Voget does state, however, that functionalists changed the way in which anthropologists began to study cultures and cultural life, with the rise of female anthropologists such as Ruth Benedict and Margaret Mead leading the way in new areas of study. Benedict became famous for her writing on *Patterns of Culture* (Benedict 1934) and Mead for her fieldtrips to study different aspects of culture, such as *Growing Up in New Guinea* (Mead 1930), *Coming of Age in Samoa* (Mead 1928) and *New Lives for Old: Cultural Transformation—Manus, 1928–1953* (Mead 1956).

These two women, who were colleagues and good friends (Lapsley 1999), remain influential to the debates on what is culture and how we can understand what it means to live in a different world through looking at unique cultures. Mead, in the preface to her 1973 edition of the book *Coming of Age in Samoa*, states that when she first wrote the book following her time living in Samoa:

> the very idea of culture was new to the literate world. The idea that our every thought and movement was a product not of race, not of instinct, but derived from the society within which an individual was reared, was new and unfamiliar (p. xxv).

She makes it clear that culture, as she saw it, did not prescribe to the thinking of many scientists at the time with regards to how people behave and what causes them to do certain things, in particular that they considered these due to the race of a person. Race and culture have a long history of debate (Donald & Rattansi 1992) but although I was very tempted to develop an additional aspect of debate to this chapter, unfortunately this will have to wait until another time.

The differences between these two separate 'schools of thought' of Malinowski and Radcliffe-Brown, noted above, will become visible in later chapters when we look at how modern-day ethnographers and anthropologists have researched various cultures or aspects of cultural life. (Given the main focus of the book and what we can realistically cover in the space allowed, for those wishing to gain more detail of this development of the discipline of anthropology, as well as the race and culture debates, additional reading can be found at the end of the chapters.)

Other definitions that we will be returning to again in other chapters are those by Professor Madeline Leininger, a nurse anthropologist from the USA and Cecil Helman, a renowned author and professor of medical anthropology. Leininger has become known for her work on developing a field of nursing called transcultural nursing, which given its relationship to the anthropological concept of culture will also be discussed in Chapter 2.

Leininger's definition of culture, for example, includes elements of Tylor's in relation to the idea of an accumulation of aspects of life over time: '*Culture is the learned and transmitted knowledge about a particular culture with its values, beliefs, rules of behaviour and lifestyle practices that guides a designated group in their thinking and actions in patterned ways*' (Leininger 1978, p. 491).

Whilst Helman (2007, p. 2) states that:

> Culture is ... a set of guidelines (both explicit and implicit) ... that an individual inherits as a member of a particular society and that tell[s] them how to view the world and learn how to experience it emotionally, and how to behave in it in relation to other people, to supernatural forces and gods, and to the natural environment. It also provides them with a way of transmitting these guidelines to the next generation – by the use of symbols, language, art and ritual. To some extent, culture can be seen as an inherited 'lens' through which the individual perceives and understands the world that he inhabits and learns how to live within it.

The issue of acquiring a set of guidelines which are either learnt, inherited or transmitted through a wide range of activities, behaviour and beliefs is reflected in both these definitions, and also to some extent in Tylor's. An interesting continuation of Helman's view of culture, and one worth expanding on for the purpose of exploring meaning in later chapters, is that culture could be viewed as:

> an inherited 'lens' through which the individual perceives and understands the world that he inhabits and learns how to live within it. Growing up within any society is a form of enculturation, whereby the individual slowly acquires the cultural 'lens' of that society. Without such a shared perception of the world, both the cohesion and continuity of any human group would be impossible' (Helman 2007, p. 2).

These definitions and viewpoints will be particularly relevant when we look at nursing as a culture or nurses as a cultural group, and whether they can be classed as a main culture in their own right or are more a subculture in the wider field of health care organisations and culture. These issues are fundamental to our developing an understanding of the anthropology of nursing, and of how anthropology for nursing can support our understanding of how nurses work and 'live' within their professional boundaries.

Anthropology and nursing

In researching widely for writing this book I had considered that most of the literature linking nursing and anthropology had begun in the 1970s in the USA with the work of Professor Madeline Leininger (1970) and her book entitled *Nursing and Anthropology: Two Worlds to Blend*. I was surprised to find, however, that there had been publications in the 1960s by Dr Mary Noble (1964) in the UK that discussed the relationship of one with the other. Dr Noble worked at the first Nursing Studies Unit at Edinburgh University, which she stated was placed in the Faculty of Social Sciences which encouraged the links between nursing and social anthropology. Her paper offers not only an insight into her view of nurses in relation to anthropology but also research where she believed that nurses should not engage in this work without a '*rigorous training in research theory and methods*' (p. 160).

She made a strong case for how social anthropology could support nursing research in '*investigating the role of the nurse in the community and in hospital*', in particular in the community nursing setting, that of '*the care of the child, of the aged and of those suffering from mental ill-health*'.

An interesting perspective she makes on the debate between those seeking 'quantitative data' and the social anthropologist who she sees uses techniques of 'participant observation and informal interviewing' is that the social anthropologist is often criticised for not using more of the former. She points out, however, in relation to this view that in fact:

> the anthropologist is primarily interested in the investigation of the content of social relationships and of the functioning of systems of relationships in terms of compatibility of role expectations and convergence towards the values of the 'whole'. These are questions which are less amenable to counting than to other, more qualitative methods of study (p. 163).

In relation to what Dr Noble sees as the relationship between nursing and social anthropology, however, she believed that '*social scientists should be encouraged to undertake nursing studies*' – as they, in her words, would '*bring to the situation an approach which is not coloured by questions of emotion or of efficiency*' (p. 161).

This could be considered in fact the beginning of a debate in nursing and, indeed, in other fields, where 'being of the culture' itself and an 'insider' cannot in fact offer an unbiased perspective of one's own culture if studied by someone from that culture itself – i.e. the emic and etic debate – and should one be able to objectively undertake research or an ethnographic study of one's own culture (see Chapter 3)?

She also highlights a number of studies where she sees that '*an anthropological viewpoint is well demonstrated*' and these will be discussed in Chapter 3 which focuses on anthropology, research and ethnography in nursing research. One example is Salisbury's (1962) *Structures of Custodial Care*, which is: An Anthropological Study of a State Mental Hospital. He offers an invaluable insight and discussion of the role he chose as an 'outsider' anthropologist who needed to be able to move about in a strange environment without causing too much disturbance of the field, in order to gain an insight into the world of both patients and staff.

Osborne in 1969, writing from the USA, focuses his position on making parallels between 'the anthropological method and nursing theory', and in particular how both focus on the 'holistic' viewpoint, namely that:

> The commitment of the nursing profession and nurses to total patient care parallel the anthropological tradition of the 'holistic' study of man. This conceptualisation of 'total patient care' is a generalising principle which gives form to nursing studies and nursing practice as the anthropological conceptualisation of 'the study of man' gives form and direction to anthropology (Osborne 1969, p. 252).

Following an exploration and consideration of nursing and health care, alongside anthropology and fieldwork, he concludes that anthropology can indeed be of value to developing 'nursing science' but at the same time nursing can also *be of value to anthropology*' (p. 255). Another major supporter of this view was Professor Madeline Leininger, who is identified as a nurse anthropologist working in the USA. A paper published first in its own right (Leininger 1967) and later reprinted in one of her books (Leininger 1978) outlined her initial ideas and direction that she thought should be important for nurses in order to care for people from different cultures.

From her early work and her doctorate studies she become famous for her development of a model framework that is meant to support nurses caring for patients from different cultures, and by which to identify their individual health care needs. The main focus of her anthropological interests and her work was centred on the culture concept which she made the most important and central issue of the transcultural nursing movement in nursing education, practice and research. Her work (Leininger 1967) led to the publishing of her ideas and theories in *Nursing and Anthropology: Two Worlds to Blend* (1970) which then developed into her 'Theory of culture care diversity and universality' (Leininger 1991) and what has become know as Leininger's Sunrise Model because of the way the nursing model is structured.

We will return in Chapter 2 to look at her views about culture and because it has in fact led to the development of a field of nursing now known as Transcultural Nursing (TCN). This has led to an explosion of articles and books, as well as the development of a specific TCN journal on this topic, as well as developments in cultural competence and care as it relates to this notion of universality of cultures and the importance on their health and illness belief systems.

Transcultural nursing also has its critics (Bruni 1988; Mulholland 1994; Gustafson 2005; Gray & Thomas 2006) and although culture is an important concept in this book I do not intend to focus on its use in a narrow way, such as in transcultural nursing models where individual cultures are reduced to looking at them as homogenous wholes and where in their use they have become prescriptive frameworks for assessment of that culture without taking account of individuals as such. Bruni (1988), for example, in her conclusion regarding the need to ensure effective care for all people, states the following:

> Transcultural theory, a framework which seeks to address the health care issues of diverse ethnic groups is one such development, however critical analysis suggests that its application may well reinforce the very problem of paternalist and ethnocentric care it seeks to address (p. 31).

Wilkins (1993) in her review of the literature at that time on transcultural nursing concluded something similar, in that:

> Culture is not a static but a dynamic process, and, even within a particular culture, the experience of the individual varies and changes with time (p. 609) and that: Therefore there could well be a danger in discussing culture-specific nursing care. This may divert attention away from the uniqueness of the Individual (p. 609).

There is, of course, much more to the debate on the value of transcultural nursing as it has developed from that first Leininger theory, and I would be remiss, given its stated origins as being related to a fusion between nursing and anthropology, to not include some reference to it, but essentially its principles have remained static and have not allowed for any major development, other than to add more and more cultures and communities to the list of those already written about by others. In the wider global nursing community, this model has mainly been used in the USA where it originated , unlike in the UK with the work of Papadopoulos et al. (1998) where cultural awareness has become a starting point and Ramsden's (2002) unique cultural safety nursing framework which also begins with cultural awareness as a starting point to achieving a level of cultural safety and an acknowledgement of the client in defining their own care. She also stresses the point that '*culture is dynamic and mobile and changes according to time, individuals and groups*' (Ramsden 2002, p. 111).

My own beliefs about how culture can be framed in nursing can be seen in the latest edition of a book on cultural awareness (Holland 2017) where I view the importance of a need initially for a broad awareness of cultural values and beliefs of individuals and communities and not a promoted need for nurses to have culture-specific knowledge of individual cultures to deliver care as it is with many transcultural nursing theorists. It is of course important to know some key issues specific to some cultures, for example about health and illness beliefs as they impact on nursing and medical care and especially in areas where there are members of specific communities who will come into regular contact with health professionals (see Shepherd et al. 2019 for different views). However, assessing nurses as culturally competent in nursing patients in aspects of that culture will require a major cultural shift in both education and practice.

I am, however, conscious that nurses need some framework to enable those they care for from any cultural group to be individually assessed rather than homogenously. The most important issue in terms of anthropology and nursing, though, is how that major concept of culture is not only defined but then used in nursing work and care to ensure that cross-cultural issues such as race, ethnicity and gender are not omitted from the discourse. This was an issue raised also in Shepherd et al.'s (2019) study.

Nursing as a 'professional culture' is, overall, omitted from the dialogue in transcultural nursing, although Leininger did write about nursing as a culture/subculture in her earlier work. This is discussed in Chapter 2.

In recent years, in a doctorate study on the topic of a critical analysis of 'Cultural Care in Nursing', Seaton (2010) offered her assessment of the literature critiquing the transcultural nursing literature and what it was based on and although this work will be discussed as it relates to an understanding and use of the concept of culture in more depth in Chapter 2, it is relevant in view of all the other authors' viewpoints pre-dating this study to highlight these findings here:

The collective findings of a critique of Transcultural Nursing, from Seaton (2010):

> *Nursing authors over the last two decades have identified significant limitations in the process of developing cultural understanding in nursing and, in particular, transcultural nursing. These authors have collectively isolated certain presumptions within notions of 'culture' and nursing care that are apparent in transcultural nursing. Together the critiques of Leininger's theory embody the following concerns that transcultural nursing theory:*
>
> - *Is largely ethnocentric;*
> - *Is primarily constructed around ethnicity as the sole issue of concern;*

- *Is positivist and reductionist, leading to a mechanistic description of ethnic groups and of the nurse's interactions with those patients, who are potentially much more complex than currently conceptualised;*
- *Constitutes a doctrine at risk of inferring cultural imposition whereby it encourages nurses to bracket out the diverse reality of cultures;*
- *Avoids issues around the socially constructed nature of culture;*
- *Isolates engagements with nurses within the presumed vacuum of an individual-to-individual context;*
- *Fails to adequately address historically driven social practices, which are embedded in exclusionary and oppressive practices within the context of healthcare;*
- *Offers a model whereby the patient is absent from the voices that constitute the discourse.*
- *Whilst they are pivotal to its construction, they have a place only as 'objects of study'. They do not have a voice in either the design or the assessment of the outcome of care as being either culturally appropriate or competent (Seaton 2010, p. 49).*

Once Leininger began to promote her work through multiple publications, other authors also began to focus on the relationship between nursing and anthropology, such as Chrisman (1982), McKenna (1984), Brink (1984), Doughtery & Tripp-Reimer (1985; 1990), Morse (1988), Dobson (1991), Mulhall (1994; 1996), DeSantis (1994), Holden & Littlewood (1991) and Mahoney & Engebretson (2000). We can consider some of their important positions on this relationship but it is important to note that all these views were specific to both international context and heath care, as well as to different time periods in the development of nursing as a profession in various countries. We will see the impact of these throughout the book.

Chrisman (1982) offers a very interesting perception of nursing being a very practice-based profession '*with a socially sanctioned and therefore morally experienced clinical or service mandate*', whereas anthropology did not, and because of this the teaching of 'anthropological understandings' to nurses '*must be translated by the anthropologist so they are relevant to patient care*' (p. 117). He then offers a very insightful introduction to his teaching of the subject to nurses in a School of Nursing as well as the challenges involved. His conclusion was, however, that '*a biomedical conceptual framework is prevalent and persuasive*' despite the developments he and colleagues had been able to make in the school. It is evident from reading the paper that his teaching at the time focused on a cross-cultural approach to nursing and anthropology and that 'anthropology for nursing' teaching emerged. The expectations of students undertaking this unique course made this clear: '*by the end of this course, the cross-cultural students have begun to perceive the value of anthropological concepts for nursing practice and to synthesize anthropology and nursing to achieve their goals in research and clinical practice*'.

McKenna (1984) focused her paper on the issues of anthropology in nursing and nursing in anthropology. Her conclusions were that '*signs of an integration of nursing in anthropology are not as evident as are studies on the application of anthropological methods in nursing research and the adaptation of anthropological concepts in nursing practice*' (p. 427). This focus is not unlike the difference outlined for this book where we have anthropology for nursing and anthropology of nursing, also identified by Holden & Littlewood (1991), but interestingly as we will discover in Chapter 3 the use of anthropological research methods (such as interviews and participant and non-participant observations) only in nursing research studies, and the adoption of the term ethnographic research as the origin in these studies, has in fact created a dissonance with the way in which the actual philosophy of the methodology steeped in anthropology is being misused.

My understanding of the paper by Brink (1984) is that of presentation of the value that anthropology has for nursing, through being taught to nurses, presenting what knowledge is required by nurses for them to care for patients, what contribution nursing has made to anthropology and most importantly for any discussion is the idea of the nurse as a culture broker between nursing and anthropology. For the purpose of new discussion I intend to briefly focus on this last issue of the nurse as culture broker. Brink identifies this role as being those '*specialists who can demonstrate by their teaching and writing the applicability of anthropological theory and method to the professional problems nursing faces*' (p. 110) and that '*simply reading an ethnography does not provide sufficient preparation to enable the health professional to use the information effectively.*' It is evident from further reading that her interpretation remains focused on seeing nurses as dealing with different cultural groups and then focusing on '*those aspects of the culture that directly influence health/illness behaviour and tradition*' (p. 111). There follows further consideration of what could be important for nurses through looking at physical anthropology, social anthropology, psychological anthropology and cultural anthropology. She considers nurse anthropologists as interpreting culture concepts. Her explanation of the debate between Leininger and others about who should or should not be entitled to be called a nurse anthropologist by virtue of different academic qualifications led her to state that:

> In the end, the definition of who is, and who is not a nurse anthropologist is one of self definition, regardless of degrees and diplomas. Individuals who call themselves, and see their professional orientation as nurse anthropologists, are nurse anthropologists (p. 131).

In the UK this drive for recognition as nurse anthropologists has not been so predominant in the literature, and not until Holden & Littlewood (1990) reported on an initial workshop which had taken place in 1986 aimed at developing '*new insights into nursing as a topic of anthropological study*' with further workshops to look at anthropology of nursing, did the issue take on a possible future direction for UK nurses working alongside medical professionals, sociologists, anthropologists and others. However, for whatever reason this drive to develop a relationship did not materialise into any major development but most importantly there arose from the workshop the Holden & Littlewood (1991) book which is still cited and has become the main text to illustrate anthropology for nursing through a number of chapters used as international cases.

From my perspective it is a starting point for defining what anthropology of nursing might be. Their definition of what it could be focuses on the following:

> For an anthropologist who is not a nurse by training, nursing provides an ethnographic field to be studied like any other. It has its own esoteric language, symbolic systems and collective identity-features which define the traditional anthropological areas of study. The social anthropologist is concerned with documenting and analysing the rites and practices of this group as s(he) might any other (Holden & Littlewood 1991).

They clearly see nursing as an ethnographic field – or if we look at ethnographic studies, a nursing culture or social group in its own right which anyone can study anthropologically. In Chapter 2 we will be exploring this concept of nursing as both profession and practice viewed as a field which can be studied from an anthropological perspective.

Anthropology for nursing is more akin to that definition of culture underpinning trans-cultural nursing where principles from anthropology can be used to help nurses understand how cultures live and believe and also how some issues can help us understand how to care for patients. For example, an understanding of how and why different cultures create body tattoos or piercings could throw a light onto why others in very different cultures, or what may be called subcultures, undertake to do the same. How different societies live in various kinship groups is also an important aspect of life from anthropological studies which can help nurses relate to experiences outside of their normal social systems.

Dougherty & Tripp-Reimer (1985) focus their review paper on four very important issues that we will discuss in various chapters. These are:

a   The contributions of nursing to medical anthropology,
b   the influence anthropology has had on nursing,
c   the differences between the interface of nursing and anthropology and that of medicine and anthropology, and
d   reasons that these differences have not been a focus in medical anthropology (p. 219)

It is not my intention to focus on all these issues as it is an incredibly detailed paper. However, some insights will be offered here and others in later chapters. The first and I think most important is their statement that the relationship between nursing and medicine has often been misunderstood, and that nursing is not a category within medicine as applied to anthropological studies. They make the point that *'there is considerable overlap in the contribution of each profession to client health, because all health professionals are generally concerned with the mental and physical well-being of clients'*. They then differentiate between them stating that medicine is more concerned with disease, or individuals and their 'bodies in disease', whereas nursing focuses more on the illness as experienced by the person because that is what clients are concerned with (p. 220). They do offer an interesting option that: *'nursing uses the model of illness and the model of disease and mediates the two'*, but are clear that the focus of their work will depend on the individual circumstance as related to their patient's (client's) health at any given time. An example could be seen as the dominance of the medical model (focus on disease) in situations such as a cardiac arrest or the reverse in situations such as chronic health issues (focus on illness experience).

Dougherty and Tripp-Reimer's chapter in *Medical Anthropology* (Johnson & Sargent 1990) stresses again the issues of difference between nursing and biomedicine in relation to anthropological studies, and they state that *'anthropologists are recognising slowly that nurses mediate the biomedical and client orientations'* (Dougherty & Tripp-Reimer 1990, p. 175), but also point out that because *'nurses operate within two models, the nursing role is more difficult to define'*. The overall concepts explored, however, had already been addressed in their 1985 article.

Mulhall (1994) offers a view of anthropology in relation to the development of transcultural nursing theories and models mainly in the USA by focusing her deliberations on *'anthropology in or for nursing'* (p. 35). She made it clear that like Holden & Littlewood (1991) she saw that *'the anthropology of nursing embraces the study of the socio-cultural features which define nursing and its practices, traditions and rituals'*; and that a possible research example to illustrate this *'might include, for example, an exploration of the symbolic and social meaning associated with a nurse's uniform'* as seen in Holden (1991). My own research (Holland 1993) pursued this approach in exploring nursing culture for the existence of rituals.

This view is specifically the one taken in this book, where the anthropology of nursing becomes the main focus, as does a social/cultural anthropology perspective in relation to culture. Mulhall's evaluation of the use of culture in transcultural nursing will be explored further in Chapter 2 as it is, like the work of Seaton (2010), central to the understanding of culture and cultural concepts that we are using in this book.

In her 1996 paper Mulhall returns to the same discussion but this time asks the question: *Anthropology, nursing and midwifery: A natural alliance*? She considers the issue of natural alliance through a consideration of their professional backgrounds and the way in which research is developing and that both nursing and midwifery '*share with anthropology a commitment to the interpretative or naturalistic paradigms*' (p. 631) (see also Chapter 3). She offers, however, 'cautionary notes' for both professions in their use in particular of the anthropological concept of culture. She clearly cautions its use in the way transcultural nursing was developing in the USA especially where culture is seen as static, reflecting its basis in American anthropology (p. 635).

De Santis (1994) offers us an insight into how to make '*anthropology clinically relevant to nursing care*', and her explanation is based on her premise that:

> Transcultural nursing is generally seen as the interface between anthropology and nursing. A prime objective of transcultural nursing has been the translation of concepts from anthropology and nursing into the nursing process to guide a culturally informed clinical practice (p. 707).

There are elements of her paper that I find contradictory in relation to what she sees as transcultural nursing and anthropology, and she offers I think a very different view of how anthropological concepts can help nurses deliver culturally appropriate care but not so narrow a view as some of the other transcultural nursing theories. I will offer here a very interesting concept that she puts forward around '*multiple cultural contexts and clinical realities*' (p. 709), and one that I have used when explaining the importance of what nurses need to consider when meeting and caring for a patient in any health care context (Holland 2017). This is what she wrote:

> Nurses who understand the concept of dual ethnocentrism view each nurse–patient encounter as an interaction of a minimum of three cultures. One culture is founded on the nurse's professional knowledge, based on the precepts of biomedicine, the beliefs, values and world view of nursing, and the nurse's personal values, beliefs and practices. The second culture is grounded in the patient's interpretation of the scope and abilities of biomedicine, based upon their life experiences with health and illness and their personal values, beliefs and practices. The third culture is the context in which the nurse–patient encounter takes place, e.g. an institution, agency, community or family setting (p. 709).

As De Santis (1994) stated, this was only a minimum of three different kinds of culture, all three of which, given that this was written in 1994, have some place in engaging nurses in exploring their own nursing culture as it relates to that of the patient and the clinical context or environment in which the nursing encounter takes place.

I believed, however, that she could have made that four cultures, and that the additional one should have been the nurse's own personal culture and beliefs outside that of a nursing culture. The other culture, of course, which could have an impact on this nurse–patient encounter and indeed could have an equivalent, is that of medicine or the biomedical culture of the doctor, but that is, for the purposes of this discourse, external to the nurse–patient encounter.

The danger with using any kind of 'explanatory model' or framework for both understanding the patient's health and illness beliefs and how to care for a patient is that it can become prescriptive of course, but sometimes there is a balance to be made to enable student nurses in particular to learn that these various cultures co-exist in their caring for patients in different contexts.

My rationale for including this fourth culture was to be able to engage the student in considering how their nursing culture worked in practice but that they brought to that nursing culture their own external personal culture and beliefs which could at times conflict with their developing professional culture. This interesting view of the multiple encounters has led to some very important discussions with student nurses concerning issues such as race, ethnicity and gender, including exploration of power relationships in and between all four cultures in the nurse–patient encounter. The important issue as Mulhall (1996) cautions is that none of these cultural encounters can be seen as static, because each nurse–patient encounter is different as is the same nurse–patient encounter at different times of the day.

Conclusion

So what have I learnt from exploring the literature on the relationship between nursing and anthropology? The first issue of course has to be that there is no clear body of evidence of anthropology or an anthropological lens that could support nursing as such and especially nursing as a culture. The second issue is that the main area where we can see anthropology of nursing topics, is through the lens of ethnography or ethnographic research which offers us an examination of topics such as rituals, death (in nursing homes and hospices), time and space in a hospice or simply the use of ethnography as a research methodology to explore an organisational culture. Thirdly, there is a need for the development of a definition of what we mean by an anthropology of nursing, so that there is at least an opportunity to stimulate debate. I have therefore made an attempt to do this and am offering two possible definitions for nursing anthropology, in order that, once the book is published, colleagues can engage in a discussion of whether either of these meets their view or we can set them aside and develop another. I found one definition of medical anthropology of particular value in beginning to think about the body of knowledge and subfield of anthropology that we could attribute in the same way to nursing anthropology. I have set it in context:

Definition of medical anthropology

Given that nurses co-exist with the medical and other health professions within the boundaries of various health care environments it is important to look at how anthropology related to medicine in particular impacts on the nursing profession and its work. Medical anthropology is one of the biggest subfields in anthropology and this definition by Pool & Geissler (2005) offers a broad overview of its content and context: '*Medical anthropology describes, interprets and critically approaches the relationships between culture, behaviour, health and disease, and places health and illness in the broader context of cultural, social, political and historical processes*' (p. 29).

Here are two possible definitions of nursing anthropology based on extensive reading for this book as well as consideration of how it could possibly align with that of medical anthropology as seen above, but ensuring the centrality of what is nursing and nursing culture. Before researching and reading for this book I found it difficult to believe that there was a way to bring together some of the available evidence for making a case for a body of knowledge that could be attributed to nursing anthropology.

Nursing anthropology: definition 1

Nursing anthropology focuses on describing the nature of the nursing profession as a major cultural group set within the context of past, present and future health care. It considers this a field where relationships between nurses, patients and others are played out in terms of cultural, social, political and historical agendas. The central focus of the nurse's role is the patient, and an understanding of their social and cultural context is reflected in the role that nurses play in ensuring their well-being through nursing as care work. This nursing work is set within various temporal, organisational and spatial contexts which are also essential to view through an anthropological lens.

Nursing anthropology: definition 2

Nursing anthropology focuses on describing the nature of the nursing profession as a major cultural group that exists within various communities of practice in health care contexts. These communities exist as fields to be studied through an anthropological lens, encompassing the nurse as the main member of the culture whose focus of existence revolves around care work as nursing. This nursing work is set within various temporal, spatial and organisational contexts which are also rich fields for exploring the nature of this unique cultural group.

I do not see this chapter, nor the book, as an end, because it is for others after reading its content to further the exploration of what anthropology of nursing – or rather nursing anthropology – is. The definitions above are to be considered in supporting the exploration.

References

A Lady Volunteer (1856) *Eastern Hospitals and English Nurses*, 3rd Edition, Hurst & Blackett Publishers, London. Reprinted in the BiblioLife Reproduction Series.
Benedict R (1934) *Patterns of Culture*, Houghton Mifflin Company, Boston. 1st Marriner Book Edition 2005.
Benedict R (1946) The Chrysanthemum and the Sword, Houghton Mifflin Company, Boston. Reprinted 1989.
Best O & Fredericks B (2014) *Yatdjuligan: Aboriginal and Torres Strait Islander Nursing and Midwifery Care*, Cambridge University Press, Melbourne.
Boas F (1962) *Anthropology and Modern Life*, Greenwood Press, Connecticut, US.
Brink P J (1984) Key issues on nursing and anthropology. In J L Ruffini (ed), *Advances in Medical Social Science*, 107–146, Vol. 2, Gordon & Breach, New York.
Bruni N (1988) A cultural analysis of transcultural theory, *The Australian Journal of Advanced Nursing*, 5(3), March–May, 26–32.
Bueno C F (2012) *Socio-Anthro: Sociology and Anthropology*, CreateSpace Independent Publishing Platform.

Bullough B & Bullough V L (1964) *The Emergence of Modern Nursing*, Macmillan, New York.

Chrisman N J (1982) Anthropology in nursing: An exploration of adaptation. In N J Chrisman and T W Maretzki (ed), *Clinically Applied Anthropology*, 117–140, D Reidel Publishing Co, Dordecht, Holland.

De Santis L (1994) Making anthropology clinically relevant to nursing care, *Journal of Advanced Nursing*, 20, 707–715.

Dobson S (1991) *Transcultural Nursing*, Scutari Press, London.

Donald J & Rattansi A (1992) (eds) *'Race' Culture and Difference*, Sage, London.

Dougherty M C & Tripp-Reimer T (1985) The interface of nursing and anthropology, *Annual Review of Anthropology*, 14, 219–241.

Dougherty M & Tripp-Reimer T (1990) Nursing and anthropology. In T M Johnson & C F Sargent (eds), *Medical Anthropology*, 174–186, Praeger, New York.

Eriksen A (2015) The authority of professional roles, *Journal of Social Philosophy*, 46(3), 373–391.

Geertz C (1973) *The Interpretation of Cultures*, Basic Books, New York.

Gourley J (2004) *Florence Nightingale and the Health of the Raj*, Routledge, Oxford.

Gray D P and Thomas D J (2006) Critical reflections on culture in nursing, *Journal of Cultural Diversity*, 13(2), 76–82.

Gustafson D L (2005) Transcultural nursing theory from a critical cultural perspective. *Advances in Nursing Science*, Jan–Mar, 28(1), 2–16.

Hagey R (1988) Retrospective on the culture concept. In J M Morse (ed), *Recent Advances in Nursing: Issues in Cross-Cultural Nursing*, 1–10, Churchill Livingstone, Edinburgh.

Helman C (2007) *Culture, Health and Illness*, 5th Edition, Hodder Arnold, London.

Hodder I (1998) The interpretation of documents and material culture. In N K Denzin & Y S Lincoln (eds), *Collecting and Interpreting Qualitative Materials*, 110–129, Sage, Thousand Oaks, CA.

Holden P (1991) Colonial sisters: Nurses in Uganda. In P Holden & J Littlewood (1991) *Anthropology and Nursing*, 67–83, Routledge, London.

Holden P & Littlewood J (1990) Preface. In P Holden & J Littlewood (1991) *Anthropology and Nursing*, Routledge, London.

Holden P & Littlewood J (1991) *Anthropology and Nursing*, Routledge, London.

Holland C K (1993) An ethnographic study of nursing culture as an exploration for determining the existence of a system of ritual, *Journal of Advanced Nursing*, 18, 1461–1470.

Holland K (2017) *Cultural Awareness in Nursing and Health Care. An Introductory Text*, 3rd Edition, Routledge, London.

Huch R K (1985) The National Association for the Promotion of Social Science: Its contribution to Victorian health reform, 1857–1886. *Albion*, 17(3), 279–299. doi:10.2307/4048958

Johnson T M & Sargent C F (eds) (1990) *Medical Anthropology: Contemporary Theory and Method*, Greenwood Press, Connecticut.

Lapsley H (1999) *Margaret Mead and Ruth Benedict: The Kinship of Women*, University of Massachusetts Press, Amherst.

Lavenda R H & Schultz E A (2010) *Core Concepts in Cultural Anthropology*, 4th Edition, McGraw-Hill, New York.

Leininger M (1967) The culture concept and its relevance to nursing, *The Journal of Nursing Education*, 27–37.

Leininger M (1970) *Nursing and Anthropology: Two Worlds to Blend*, John Wiley & Sons, New York.

Leininger M (1978) *Transcultural Nursing: Concepts, Theories and Practices*. John Wiley & Sons, New York. Republished in 1990.

Leininger M (1991) Theory of culture care diversity and universality, *National League for Nursing*, Washington.

Mahoney J S & J Engebretson (2000) The interface of anthropology and nursing guiding culturally competent care in psychiatric nursing, *Archives of Psychiatric Nursing*, 14(4), 183–190.

Malinowski B (1954) *Argonauts of the Western Pacific*, Routledge and Kegan Paul, London. (Published originally in 1922.)

McKenna M (1984) Anthropology and nursing: The interaction between fields of inquiry, *Western Journal of Nursing Research*, 6(4) 423–431.

Mead M (1928) *Coming of Age in Samoa*. Republished in 2001 by Harper Perennial, New York.

Mead M (1930) *Growing Up in New Guinea: A Comparative Study of Primitive Education*, William Morrow, New York.

Mead M (1956) *New Lives for Old: Cultural Transformation—Manus, 1928–1953*, William Morrow, New York.

Monaghan J & Just P (2000) *Social & Cultural Anthropology: A Short Introduction*, Oxford University Press, Oxford.

Morse J M (1988) *Issues in Cross-cultural Nursing (Recent advances in nursing)*, Churchill Livingstone, Edinburgh.

Mulhall A (1994) Anthropology: A model for nursing, *Nursing Standard*, 8(31), 35–38.

Mulhall A (1996) Anthropology, nursing and midwifery: A natural alliance? *International Journal of Nursing Studies*, 33(6) 629–637.

Mulholland J (1994) Nursing, humanism and transcultural theory: The 'bracketing-out' of reality, *Journal of Advanced Nursing*, 22(3), 442–449.

Navy Military Press (2009) Description of content of *Eastern Hospitals and English Nurses* (https://www.naval-military-press.com/product/eastern-hospitals-and-english-nurses-the-narrative-of-twelve-m onths-experience-in-the-hospitals-of-koulali-and-scutari/).

Nightingale F (1865) Note on the aboriginal races of Australia: a paper read at the annual meeting of the National Association for the Promotion of Social Science, held at York, September, 1864. Emily Faithfull, printer and publisher in ordinary to Her Majesty, Victoria Press, London (https://croakey.org/wp-content/uploads/2017/10/Nightingale1865.-NotesonAboriginalRaces.pdf, accessed 6 May 2019).

Noble M (1964) Social anthropology and nursing, *International Journal of Nursing Studies*, 1, 159–163.

Osborne O H (1969) Anthropology and nursing: Some common traditions and interests, *Nursing Research*, May–June, 18(3), 251–253.

Papadopoulos I, Tilki M and Taylor G (1998) *Transcultural Care: A Guide for Health Care Professionals*, Quay Books, Wilts.

Pool R & Geissler W (2005) *Medical Anthropology*, Open University Press, Maidenhead.

Radcliffe-Brown A R (1935) On the concept of function in social science, *American Anthropologist*, 37, 394–402.

Ramsden I M (2002) *Cultural Safety and Nursing Education in Aotearoa and Te Waipounamu*, Unpublished PhD study, Victoria University of Wellington, New Zealand (https://croakey.org/wp-content/uploads/2017/08/RAMSDEN-I-Cultural-Safety_Full.pdf).

Salisbury R F (1962) *Structures of Custodial Care: An Anthropological Study of a State Mental Hospital*, University of California Press, Berkeley and Los Angeles.

Seaton L P (2010) *Cultural Care in Nursing: A Critical Analysis*, Unpublished PhD study, University of Technology, Sydney (https://opus.lib.uts.edu.au/bitstream/2100/1130/4/02Whole.pdf; https://www.researchgate.net/publication/265496391_Cultural_care_in_nursing_A_critical_analysis, accessed 30 April 2019).

Sera-Shriar E (2014) What is armchair anthropology? Observational practices in 19th-century British human sciences, *History of Human Sciences*, 27(2), 26–40.

Shepherd S M, Willis-Esqueda C, Newton D, Sivasubramaniam D & Paradies Y (2019). The challenge of cultural competence in the workplace: Perspectives of healthcare providers, *BMC Health Services Research*, 19(1), 135. doi:10.1186/s12913-019-3959-7

Stocking G W (1968) *Race, Culture and Evolution: Essays in the History of Anthropology*, University of Chicago Press, Chicago.

Tylor E B (1871) *Primitive Culture*, London.

Van Maanen J (1988) *Tales of the Field: On Writing Ethnography*, University of Chicago Press, Chicago.

Vogel E F (1989) Foreword. In R Benedict, *The Chrysanthemum and the Sword: Patterns of Japanese Culture*, Houghton Mifflin Company, Boston. Originally published in 1946.

Voget F W (2009) Man and culture: An essay in changing anthropological interpretation, *American Anthropologist*, New Series, 62(6), 943–965.

Wilkins H (1993) Transcultural nursing: A selective review of the literature, 1985–1991, *Journal of Advanced Nursing*, 18(4) 602–612.

Further reading

1 Boas F (1932) The aims of anthropological research, *Science*, New series, 76(183), 605–613.

2 Dingwall R, Rafferty A M & Webster R (1988) *An Introduction to Social History of Nursing*, Routledge, London.

3 Hahn R A & InhornM C (2009) *Anthropology and Public Health: Bridging Differences in Culture and Society*, 2nd Edition, Oxford University Press, Oxford.

4 Keesing R M & StrathernA J (1998) *Cultural Anthropology: A Contemporary Perspective*, 3rd Edition (hardcover), Wadsworth/Thomson Learning, USA.

5 Morse J M (ed) (1988) *Cross-Cultural Nursing Anthropological Approaches to Nursing Research*, Gordon & Breach, New York.

2

CULTURE AND NURSING

An anthropological perspective

Karen Holland

Introduction

As seen in Chapter 1 we have discerned that the concept of culture is an essential principle of anthropology, and therefore the anthropology of nursing. It is advised that for those entirely new to linking nursing and culture that you read Chapter 1 first, as there are related concepts and evidence that need to be understood in terms of anthropology.

This chapter will therefore focus on the meaning of culture as it relates to nursing (and therefore nurses) as both a profession and as work, exploring whether it meets the definition of a culture that can be explored anthropologically. (See Chapter 1 for the main definitions associated with a culture.)

I will also consider the evidence as to whether we can consider it as a culture in its own right with its own boundaries and ways of existing. In addition, and given nursing exists as both a profession and work within the wider organisational culture of health care, the two fields of education and practice as related to health care will be taken as the background in which to explore the evidence of nursing as a culture. (See also Chapter 5 and Chapter 6.)

In order to ensure that there is a commonality of understanding about the nature of nursing which is central to this book and this chapter, I will begin the narrative with an overview of what nursing is and also how it has developed over time, with a particular focus on the historical and political context of nurse education. In one respect I have already positioned myself as believing that nursing is a culture, having already undertaken a very early ethnography which concluded that nursing has at least a 'cultural system' (Holland 1993). I will, however, present what evidence there is about the development of nursing over time, as 'cultural snapshots' only so that readers can determine for themselves if this evidence is clearly visible or not. Further Reading will be given to enable readers to enhance their understanding of nursing over time.

We also know that culture is not considered '*to be a static but a dynamic process, and even within a particular culture, the experience of the individual varies and changes with time*' (Wilkins 1993, p. 609). Time has become a major theme in one way or another across many chapters in this book and is of itself another major theme within the anthropological literature. (See Chapter 4 as it relates to nursing.)

Nursing as both an occupation and profession

Nursing is an established occupation throughout the world and is clearly seen as work that involves dealing with illness and sickness in society. The belief and value systems inherent within nursing relate directly to this raison d'être, and as with any society allow nurses to deal effectively with the events occurring as an outcome of disease and sickness. Rafferty (1996, p. 1) believes that: *'Education lies at the centre of professional work and expertise and therefore occupies a pivotal position in the shaping of occupational culture and the politics of nursing.'*

If we look closely at the literature on the development of nursing as a professional occupation and nurse education in particular (they are inextricably linked through the educational journey of a student nurse's learning to become a nurse – Chapter 6) we can see that it can be examined through different periods of time in history – historical lenses or 'cultural snapshots' of the world – revealed to us through historical data, literature and empirical studies. This will only be a 'snapshot approach' to the development of nursing and it could be argued that it is easier to consider if viewed from what can be called 'the development of modern nursing' and 'modern nursing' periods in terms of historical time. There will be overlapping of ideas across these artificial boundaries as we begin to search out the key elements of a nursing culture.

Kaminski (2006) stated that *'examining culture with context and process is barren and meaningless exercise'* and offers a number of lenses through which to analyse it. A particular analogy she uses about the culture of nursing is that *'it can be compared to a kaleidoscope, a multifaceted lens that creates an unique image based on the interplay of illumination, reflection and patterns'* (p. 3).

(See Further Reading for extensive literature on the development of nursing as I will focus here only on key aspects of the culture of nursing as a profession over time.)

In terms of nursing culture these time frames are very important because we will see the changes that impact on a culture as a whole but also make visible that which remains at the core of nursing as a professional culture. Temporality is a major concept in anthropology and I will be focusing on this in more detail in Chapter 4.

The development of modern nursing: probationers, training and the status of nurses

The origins of nursing as an acceptable occupation for women in the UK emerged out of what could be argued was the idolatry of Florence Nightingale and the political drive for registration of nurses. The outcome of years of frustration with being unable to pursue her devotion to the cause of nursing saw Florence Nightingale setting up the first training school for nurses at St Thomas's Hospital in 1860 (Seymer 1960). Fifteen probationer nurses were enrolled and thus began an initial example of the future of the modern trained nurse. These new recruits (probationers) lived together in what was an early version of the Nurses' Home, a place where character building became the responsibility of women called Home Sisters. Their responsibility was the moral training of the probationers.

As more Schools of Nursing were set up there emerged a training syllabus which focused mainly on the practice duties, i.e. nursing at the bedside. This was true of the USA as well as the UK. We can now see the development of more organised nursing groups both in relation to nursing as work but also as individual intakes of probationers each year. This can be seen as the precursor of the 'set system' as discussed by Gillian MacGuire (1968) in her paper on the function of this approach.

I myself belonged to one such 'set', with its title given a numerical name according to when we commenced our nurse training. In my case this was '1967/2', and we celebrated our 50th anniversary in September 2017. In terms of the 'set' structure, this remains an established part of the nurse education system and therefore the student nurses who are recruited and enter their future profession as intakes, either once or twice a year, can also be referred to as a cohort.

One of the important consequences of this set system approach as defined by MacGuire was that:

> The hierarchy of the sets within the grade of student nurse in a hospital constitutes the sum total of the various status positions which are available. The principle on which the sets are stratified is occupational skill. The hospital attempts to give meaning to the various levels by associating them with specific skills in a graded sequence. Mobility in this system is based in the principal of 'social age'. By social age I mean the length of time the individual has been associated with the hospital (p. 280).

Those of you who are reading this section, who may be older to nursing than I am or new as in commencing in 2019, will already be thinking about how you were/are considered in your course of study, namely first years, second years and third years. Each intake of probationers, and now student nurses, were given a number which would stay with them throughout their course, but as individuals they will move each year from one to two to three, which is the final year today for most student nurses. (I will return to this idea of 'moving' from place to place in Chapter 6, as student nurses are like 'nomadic' groups moving from one clinical placement to another as well as to and from their main home base of the university.)

MacGuire (1968) then offers her view on what this system of 'social age' groups are like: where '*the set in the hospital situation can, in all seriousness, be compared to the "age set" of the anthropological monograph*' (p. 280).

She states that:

> Nursing as a social system is analogous to the Samoan age–grade structured society which Margaret Mead has described. Here the society is stratified according to age and the socialisation process is not based on an interchange between adult and child but between the age group immediately above and the one immediately below (p. 280).

So from the first probationers, then the students, in their 'sets' there is clearly the development of a hierarchy according to age (that of years in training being the most clearly visible) in that 'learning to be a nurse' context. This also remains after they succeed in their training, in the hierarchical structures within health care organisation contexts such as hospitals. Roles such as ward sister and matron, along with this grouping of individuals into sets remain, and as MacGuire explained, for example:

the presentation of prizes, the pinning of badges and the uniform decorations, epaulettes … appropriate to year groups or sub-groups within a year constitute the rites of passage of the nursing community which emphasise the group nature of the movement towards adulthood (p. 281)

See Chapter 5 for more detail.

In considering this entrance into nursing and using Macguire's views as a starting point, we can begin to see that nurses as a group become divided into student nurses and once qualified are named something else according to the group hierarchy, or in this case the wider society of nursing. We will see that this is not an isolated pattern to nurses in one country but that this pattern of student nurse grouping, moving from place to place (also recognised as 'bounded units' of clinical placements or university classrooms) has been, and remains, the normal pattern of what we could say is a student nurse subculture within the wider nursing culture.

We have seen that the ongoing development of each group of probationers was reliant on the use of the syllabus, which could be viewed also as a means whereby the 'cultural' knowledge, skills and professional and moral attitudes were enshrined for each successive generation of probationer nurses, much like a 'cultural blueprint' for existing in that specific group. This idea of the syllabus has developed now into the curriculum, which Lawton (1989), in the context of the 'national curriculum' for education in schools, sees as the way in which society generally ensures, through the vehicle of education, that what is essential to be 'passed on' to the next generation is the most appropriate aspects of the wider culture. This view can be translated into what happens in today's nursing curriculum.

Returning to the issue of where these probationers lived, the Nurses' Home, we can see the influence that religion and morality had on the early nurses. This was a closed community and ensured a 'cloistered' living, which was reminiscent, one could argue, of the life of a nun. There was an order to their lives and probationer nurses were under constant surveillance – both in their work and in their moral behaviour (Rafferty 1996). This surveillance was also seen where they carried out their nursing work, as they and the patients they cared for could be observed easily given the special structure of the wards where they mainly worked at the time. These are still called 'Nightingale wards' given that all the patients were visible at any given time, being ordered in bed sequence down each side of a ward with a nurses' station in the middle. (See http://www.king scollections.org/exhibitions/specialcollections/nightingale-and-hospital-design/flor ence-nightingale-and-hospital-design for a visual image of a ward). You could argue in sociological terms that this was like the Foucauldian 'panoptic' surveillance, where the culture that prevailed was one where ensuring order was maintained by controlling both probationer and patients (Henderson 1994; Wolf et al 2012).

Dorcy (1992, p. 634) believed that '*the two main themes of Nightingale's model for nurse training were cloisterisation and supervision.*' Cloisters serve two purposes – enclosure and exclusion, both of which could be seen in Schools of Nursing during this Nightingale period and indeed much later into the 1960s and early 1970s. The links to Goffman's work on total institutions can also be seen in this approach, where all aspects of living were not '*spatially divided off from one another*' (Dorcy 1992, p. 637). Goffman, of course, in his work called *Asylums*, which is classed by many as an ethnography (Goffman 1961), offers this explanation of what a total institution is:

All aspects of life are conducted in the same place and under the same single authority; each phase of the member's daily activity is carried on in the immediate company of a large batch of others, all of who are treated alike and required to do the same things together; all phases of the day's activities being imposed from above by a system of explicit formal rulings and a body of officials. Finally the various enforced activities are brought together into a single rational plan purportedly designed to fulfil the official aims of the institution (Goffman 1961, p. 17).

Melosh (1982, p. 49) also refers to Goffman's work in relation to how the hospital environment *'shaped the student's experience of apprenticeship and initiation'*. In particular, how:

Total institutions deliberately construct a separate social world, marked off by systematic and routine violations of 'outside' expectations. While normal social rules balance individual autonomy against the demands of social life, total institutions submerge or deny individual claims in the service of institutional goals (p. 49).

Whether we can still argue that student nurses, and indeed nurses, still inhabit these kinds of environments remains important to the exploration of whether nursing (at large as it were) is a culture, and whether the idea of institutional living and working remains an essential part of nursing today. (See Chapter 6 on the initiation of the student nurse.)

Returning to the pre-1919 period in UK nursing's history, the debate which was to begin the professionalisation of nursing had a major impact on the education and training of nurses. Mrs Bedford Fenwick and like-minded individuals began to call for a need to regulate the work of nurses and ensure that anyone calling herself a nurse was fit to bear this title. They became the pro-registration of nursing lobby. Theirs was a model for nursing based on the medical model in order to establish it as a profession with specific entry requirements and education as well as training, away from the hospital which had been central to its continuation previously. This was vehemently opposed by Florence Nightingale, who did not believe that the art of nursing could be learnt from books and lectures (Helmstader 2007). It is important to recall that this debate was also set against the emancipation of women during the late 1800s and early 1900s, with the first stage of the vote for women being the Representation of the People Act 1918:

In 1918 the Representation of the People Act was passed which allowed women over the age of 30 who met a property qualification to vote. Although 8.5 million women met this criteria, it only represented 40 per cent of the total population of women in the UK.

This was followed by the Equal Franchise Act 1928:

It was not until the Equal Franchise Act of 1928 that women over 21 were able to vote and women finally achieved the same voting rights as men. This act increased the number of women eligible to vote to 15 million.

See this Government UK website for information on these developments: http://www.parliament.uk/about/living-heritage/transformingsociety/electionsvoting/womenvote/overview/thevote/.

This push for registration heralded the debate between the apprenticeship system of training and the formal education of professional status. It also began to model itself on what was known as the 'scientific' medical profession, whilst at the same time controlling its own practice through gatekeeping and protecting the public from unsuitable nurses. The anti-registrationists argued for a non-intellectual route, which did not emulate the medical model. Florence Nightingale's philosophy related to eradicating the effects of poverty and dirt through cleanliness and 'public health' contrasted with the work of the nurse, seen as a 'dirty job' that only women with vocational interest would do (see Chapter 8).

This idea of nursing is a critical one in terms of how it is seen in different countries, such as India (Nair 2012), and also as a nursing culture. For example, body care in particular was seen as a 'dirty' task, associated with low status in both nursing and society (Lawler 1991; Somjee 1991). Contrary to this, the role of the doctor, and therefore medical culture, was seen as a higher status as doctors had their own body of knowledge based on disease and its treatment. This developed into a clear division of labour in health work (see Chapter 7) and as Rafferty (1996: 25) explained, nursing brought the *domestic hierarchy into the workplace*.

This positioning of nursing in relation to hierarchy of labour with medics, may at first seem to be unconnected to an exploration of whether nursing can be called a culture, but as we shall see in other chapters, the nature of nursing work is fundamental to both being called a profession, with all this is meant to entail, and also employment as a nurse. I offered two possible definitions of what nursing anthropology could be in Chapter 1.

I think, here, we can further consider the issue of nursing as a culture in relation to social, political and historical agendas, through that of definition 1, namely:

> Nursing anthropology focuses on describing the nature of the nursing profession as a major cultural group set within the context of past, present and future health care. It considers this a field where relationships between nurses, patients and others are played out in terms of cultural, social, political and historical agendas. The central focus of the nurse's role is the patient, and an understanding of their social and cultural context is reflected in the role that nurses play in ensuring their well-being through nursing as care work. This nursing work is set within various temporal, organisational and spatial contexts which are also essential to view through an anthropological lens.

The issue of organisational and spatial contexts of nursing during this period in history mainly focused on the hospital and the training school, which was established at this time in hospital grounds. According to Hector (1973) at St Bart's Hospital, London, *in November 1882, a three year training was introduced* and although she believed that in part this was due to the fact that *the nurse was now beginning to enlarge her sphere of work, as the surgeon and physician increased their knowledge* (p. 30), *unfortunately, it must also be admitted that the principle reason was to increase the number of staff in the wards by retaining the girls for a further year*.

She also makes a very interesting statement as regards to the length of time it took to train a nurse, that the three-year training period had been retained even in 1973, but that also probationers (student nurses) were also paid an annual wage. Often the service needs of the hospital took precedence over the training needs of the probationers (student nurses). (See Chapter 7: Nursing work within nursing culture.)

The issue of how long it takes to educate and train a nurse remains a topic of debate today, as many countries grapple with not enough registered nurses for the future.

Through these words of Hector (1973) we can begin to see a picture emerging of how nursing began to evolve into more of a cohesive structure to nursing as work and to nurses as a group of women brought together for a common cause of nursing patients in specific areas of an organisation such as a hospital (see Chapter 4). The actual decision with regards to nurse registration could be argued to be the beginning of a new phase of change in nursing culture, certainly in the UK, and there is evidence that due to external and internal developments a culture cannot be static, although its inherent way of life in terms of what makes it distinct as that culture remains (see later in this chapter).

Modern nursing: professional registration and the development of nursing

The culmination of the debate – or as Winifred Hector (1973, p. 35) in her study of the work of Mrs Bedford Fenwick called it, 'a battle' – about the registration of nurses, and therefore their regulation in the workplace, was marked by The Nurses Registration Act of 1919. The Act itself established the ability for self-regulation, which according to the professionalisation literature is one of the key elements of professional status (Volmer & Mills 1966, p. 9).

If we consider nursing as a culture, we will need to return to this debate later, as there is literature that discusses nursing as a 'professional culture' (Strouse & Nickerson 2016) which refers not to the wider anthropological view of nursing as a culture but the very specific nature of nursing as one of the professional cultures or subcultures as identified by Friedson (1986)

The probationer nurses were caught in the middle of this pursuit for professional status, as along with the untrained nursing assistants (auxiliaries) they became the main labour force in nursing patients. According to Abel-Smith (1960) the phrase student nurse first appeared in a draft Labour Party policy advocating changes in the nursing professional whereby it was suggested that there was: '*A 48-hour week, the separation of nursing schools from the hospitals and student status for probationers with proper time for study*' (p. 137).

However, this separation did not take place until the advent of what became known widely as Project 2000 (UKCC 1986) in 1989 (see Chapters 5 and 6). The regulation and registration of nurses set the scene for debates, especially in the sociological literature (Hugman 1991; Allen 2007; Traynor & Buus 2016) about whether nursing (as an occupation) was a profession and a culture in its own right as opposed to being a subculture group of the medical profession. Anthropologically, literature on both these issues has been limited. Mallidou et al. (2011) indicate in their work on 'nurse speciality subcultures and patient outcomes in acute care hospitals' that in fact many disciplines, even today, '*lag behind in exploring their own cultures and sub-cultures*' (p. 81).

At the same time that all these changes were taking place in the UK in the post registration for nurses period, there were also major changes taking place in other countries. In particular in the USA were those changes regarding the form of training that was being established, the closeness of the hospitals to schools of nursing and what Ashley (1976, p. 16) described as the 'business of apprenticeships'. This included the debate as the profession developed as to whether students were workers or learners (see Chapter 7 on nursing work and Chapter 6 on student nurse transition). Most importantly in relation to what we have discussed so far, Ashley (1976) placed her observations of the development of nursing in the USA in the context of the continued paternalism of the medical profession that had been a dominant factor for so long. Suzanne Gordon (2005) offers an insightful and innovative view of the development and work of nurses in the USA and how different issues, such as their media image and relationship to medicine, actually often undermine nurses' work and patient care.

In India, there had been the major involvement of Florence Nightingale in the history of its health care and nursing, and in particular a protracted debate and discussion with the Governor General of India in 1867 (Gourlay 2004) who had decided, following his own local work, that some of her ideas for setting up Schools of Nursing in India were not well thought out. Gourlay (2004) explores these issues and many others in relation to the impact and influence of Nightingale on both the development of nursing and the much wider issues of sanitation and public health, in what I consider to be a very important historical insight into the development of the culture of nursing in India at that point in time.

However, in India there were similar issues related to the perceived social status of female nurses in relation to the nature of nursing work (Somjee 1991; Johnson 2010) and, of course, in the UK and USA in nursing's perceived relationship to medicine as a profession (see Chapter 7).

What is important to understand in relation to the development of nursing worldwide at this time and indeed since, is that nursing is both profession and employment or work developed against a similar backdrop. This was mainly the status of the kind of work that nurses undertook, that they were women in a world where men dominated generally and one where health care was dominated by the medical profession (see Nair 2012; George 2005; Reddy 2015).

Importantly, of course, related to this latter domination was the ownership of knowledge that was centred around the health and health care of the patient. Allen (1997) illustrates this in relation to the way in which nurses and doctors work, in her article discussing ethnographic research she conducted, namely: 'The nursing-medical boundary: a negotiated order?', and the question forming the research she undertook to explore this boundary. One of the key themes arising in her findings was the fact that nurses perceived that because of their priority, i.e. 'to do nursing' (p. 505), there was only negotiation when they were not busy and that they only undertook doctor-devolved work when this was the case. Allen (1997), however, saw from her observations that this was not as clear cut as this and that *'carrying out doctor-devolved activities clearly made sense within the constraints of the work context'* (p. 505).

This related also to Svensson's (1996) idea of the 'negotiated space' that was created by doctors and nurses to enable them to work together. However, Allen (1997) concluded that, because of the dissonance between her interview accounts and her field observations (p. 516), she in fact saw *'little evidence of negotiations or inter-occupational strains on the wards'*, which led her to consider that the *'non-negotiated informal boundary-blurring was a taken for granted feature of normal nursing practice'*. Both these studies are placed in the mid-1990s, as are the work of Wicks (1998) and Davies (1995), with varied positions on this idea of negotiated boundaries between nurses and doctors. However, Allen, after undertaking further ethnographic research (Allen 2001) which considered the changing shape of nursing practice with regards to its role in the division of labour in hospital, raised a new addition to this negotiation of boundaries between these two professional groups: that of the patient's role (Allen 2001, p. 159). She concluded that one of the key issues that impacted on the development of participatory models of practice in nursing as it related to patients and their care, was the external influence of consumerism where the needs of the patients became a priority. This tended to hide much of what nurses did, either working with other team members such as medics, or the patients, to the extent that more of nurses' work became 'invisible'. We can see from this brief insight into professional boundaries, that nursing as working with others is a fundamental part of the overall changing culture that is nursing.

To understand further about the nature of this nursing culture as it is viewed within the actual work of nurses itself, requires us to look both at the actual activities that nurses undertake as part of their daily activities and also at their role in the wider context of their identity. This will be considered in Chapter 7.

Nursing as a culture and subculture: the cultural context of nursing

Before we explore the evidence that can help us to explore this view that nursing and therefore nurses have a culture and belong to a cultural group, let us remind ourselves of the definitions of what a culture is used in Chapter 1, by looking at Helman (2007):

> Culture is … a set of guidelines (both explicit and implicit) … that an individual inherits as a member of a particular society and that tell them how to view the world and learn how to experience it emotionally, and how to behave in it in relation to other people, to supernatural forces and gods, and to the natural environment. It also provides them with a way of transmitting these guidelines to the next generation – by the use of symbols, language, art and ritual. To some extent, culture can be seen as an inherited 'lens' through which the individual perceives and understands the world that he inhabits and learns how to live within it (p. 2).

So far we have looked at nursing – as a profession and as work – to set the broader context of what this is for a specific group of individuals in society called nurses. These groups of nurses can be found in global situations and given their historical development we can already see that there are certain aspects of their world that appear in every group, such as training to become a qualified nurse, the actual work of nursing and their role with sick people in various spaces such as a hospital or their status both within and without the specific society in which they exist.

In very basic terms, we can assume then by this definition above, that nurses could be viewed culturally, i.e. as having a culture which we can see from our own experiences and also from studies about the way in which they exist as small groups in various organisational spaces or countries. Also they can be viewed as the *broader family group known as Nurses* and their main role in any society, that is their undertaking of the practice of nursing work related to patients, which from an historical perspective is their raison d'être. Littlewood (1991) states this very clearly in her exploration of the mediation role of the nurse:

> Nursing is work with people who transgress certain social expectations of activity and personal responsibility: that is, individuals who are sick. It is argued that the presence of the nurse maintains the person, encapsulated, in the wider social world during this temporary state of sickness. In so doing she herself becomes an ambiguous figure. The ambiguity of the nurse centres round two functions: as an advocate on behalf of patients in a predominantly biomedical health system she mediates between lay and professional notions of distress and responsibility, and she deals with the disruption of normative time and space caused by sickness (p. 170).

We would expect, then, that nurses as cultural groups can be defined by the way that they live and exist within the broad 'family' of nursing, and that they would exhibit all the characteristics of culture as seen in the definitions above.

In 1993 I had an article published exploring the existence of a system of ritual in nursing, and before undertaking the research had to develop a framework with which to contextualise the study in terms of nursing as a culture, and then explore through an ethnographic study whether ritual existed as part of a culture.

As we have seen from Chapter 1, at the time I started the research there was very little nursing research being undertaken using ethnography as both methodology and as the written narrative. I was also very much a novice in this field as well as the anthropological context. Suominen et al. (1997) also commented that in fact '*the structures of nursing culture remain very much unknown territory and are seldom discussed either in practice or in research*' (p. 186). The study undertaken therefore must be seen in the context of what was available at the time, both in terms of nursing culture, nursing rituals and ethnographic research.

Holden & Littlewood's book highlighting some broad perspectives in anthropology and nursing was published in 1991 but did not look specifically at the use of ethnography in nursing. As a mature undergraduate student, with the support of my tutor, I went in at the deep end (see Chapter 3), both methodologically and anthropologically, and used Beals et al.'s (1977) components of a cultural system as my initial framework. They had identified five components of such a cultural system:

- A group or society consisting of a set of members
- An environment within which the membership carried out its characteristic activities
- A material culture consisting of equipment and artefacts used by the membership and including the permanent and tangible effect that past and present membership have had on the environment
- A cultural tradition representing the historically accumulated decisions of the membership or its representatives
- Human activities and behaviours emerging out of the complex interactions among the membership, the environment, the material culture and the cultural tradition

Although this had helped my understanding of the possible existence of nurses as a cultural group, this definition wasn't specific enough regarding a ritual system, which is what I wanted to search for. Through further study I found additional material concerning what requirements there were in any society's existence to make it work as a whole and turned to the work of sociologist Talcott Parsons. Parsons belonged to a group of sociologists who were known as structural functionalists, and were very interested in how social order was maintained in society. His published work, *The Social System* (Parsons 1951), he saw as '*a conceptual scheme for the analysis of social systems in terms of the action frame of reference.*' He described it as '*intended as a theoretical work in a strict sense*' and that '*naturally the value of the conceptual scheme here put forward is ultimately to be tested in terms of its usefulness in empirical research*' (p. 3).

In my own simplistic way I sought to explore whether this 'social system' theory could help me to determine whether there was a system of ritual within a nursing group context (Holland 1993).

It is important to note that Parsons made it clear that it was '*attention confined to systems of interaction of a plurality of individual actors orientated to a situation and where the system includes a commonly understood system of cultural symbols*' that he wished to focus on (p. 5). His attempt to explain the use of the word 'actor' in this theory was based on the person or an individual as a 'social object', but if the social system he theorised about was to be able to function as a whole, this also had to contain both 'physical objects' (which could be translated as meaning the physical or environmental) and *'cultural objects which are symbolic elements of the cultural tradition, ideas or beliefs, expressive symbols or value patterns'*. So his starting point rested on *'the general theory of action systems'*. Allan (2016, p. 9) states that *'the idea of society functioning as a system dependent on its parts was very much a feature of the USA and UK in the 1950's'*.

One of the major areas of Parson's work remains very much a focus of health care and in particular is the relationship between doctors and patients. Allan (2016) discusses what is known as 'the sick role' that is adopted by individuals who become ill, and where there is the belief that to adopt the outcomes of this 'sick role', such as taking time off work, it is then sanctioned by the doctor who has the power to diagnose and legitimise that the person is ill in the first place. Allan (2016, p. 12) points out, however, that when it comes to the nursing role in Parson's model: *'that the nurses had (having) the medicine key didn't mean she had power necessarily.'* This notion of power relationships between doctors and nurses can be seen in other chapters. (Please see Further Reading for Allan's explanation of Talcott Parson's work in sociological theory.)

Based on an initial understanding of what minimum requirements were necessary to meet Parson's view of society I identified the following:

- A system of communication
- An economic system
- Arrangements for socialisation of new members
- A system of authority and distribution of power
- The possibility of a system of ritual serving to maintain or increase social cohesion and to give social recognition to significant personal events such as birth, puberty, courtship, marriage and death (Holland 1993, p. 1462)

A detailed account of the research is not possible (see Holland 1993 and Chapter 5 for details about rituals in nursing) but I can offer a surface analysis of the 'cultural scene' where I undertook the ethnographic participant observation – the cultural scene being the context in which nurses undertake their occupational roles and where student nurses undertake, in 'nomadic fashion', their clinical practice experiences and learning to become nurses. In terms of the research field, this was known as a 'surgical ward' and, for the student nurses, a clinical placement. This cultural scene is based on my observations and analysis across these aspects of a society:

1. Social structures
2. Authority
3. Economic system
4. Communication
5. Socialisation
6. Rituals

As I have already stated the study could be criticised for its naivety of intellectual discourse and methodological implementation. However, there was sufficient evidence from the observations and interviews to be able to draw some conclusions, both from an emic and etic perspective. (See Chapter 3 for definitions of these.)

In a surface analysis of the cultural scene in which I undertook the ethnography, the following patterns were observed (Holland 1993) and they established the background context to determining whether any kind of ritual system existed. They formed part of the ethnographic description of the nursing culture on the observation ward.

Social structures

These were wards of a hospital created especially to 'house on a temporary or permanent basis, the sick in society'. Each ward was separated from others within the hospital building itself and allocated its own space (see Chapter 4). The whole hospital appeared to have its own organisational culture and it appeared that nearly everything that happened in the ward took place according to a set time. The patients in the ward where I was undertaking observation 'were allowed in on the basis that they had a medically diagnosed specific disordered body function which required surgical intervention' (Holland 1993, p. 1466). The domain analysis had revealed a special language and terminology associated with this intervention, which was linked to specific body parts and function. Nurses talked about patients in relation to these interventions and terminology, such as appendicectomy, amputation, prostatectomy.

Authority

This view of authority was linked to distribution of power, and could be seen in the division of labour based on rank order and experiences rather than gender. It was seen in the titles given to individuals and also the alphabetical grading awarding different nursing roles. The power distribution was associated with the way in which care was delivered, such as team nursing with named team leaders who had commensurate grade according to level of responsibility. There was also a clear differentiation between doctors and nurses on this ward and of course the patients. It seemed that the nurses became on many occasions the intermediary between the patient and the doctor. The doctors on this ward were called surgeons as they were also differentiated by name according to the kind of medicine they practiced (see Chapter 7).

Economic system

The economic system within a hospital and therefore this ward within the hospital, it could be argued, centres around 'patient work'. Those that worked on the ward had a working day which was 'organised around both "social" and clock "time"' as identified by Zerubavel (1979). Nurses appeared to undertake their nursing work in relation to the patient according to what was known as the 'off-duty rota which in reality gave information regarding time spent at work and not time away' (p. 1466). Over a 24-hour day social time was as important as 'clock time', where social time was given names such as coffee time, lunch time and meeting time, and clock time more specifically set hours of work known as 'shift time'. Examples of the latter could be 7.30am–3pm or 2pm–8pm or 8pm–8am (the night shift). This view of nurses work time of course resonated with other occupations that depended on this pattern of time to keep their business functioning. The whole hospital also operated on 'clock time' for key activities that ensured that patients (being the main function) were given the care that they needed. One example of where social time and clock time depended on each other was in relation to visiting time – whereby relatives and friends came into the ward to see the patients at set times allocated across the overall hospital. (See Chapter 4 for further explanation.)

Communication system

The nurses on the ward appeared to have their own 'nursing' language, which was evident verbally and also textually in their day-to-day writing, especially about the care they delivered to the patients. They also appeared to have a number of ways to communicate about their work and the patients in their care. They had a system of ensuring that information about patients was transferred to anyone new that came to work on the ward, especially when they changed their 'work shifts'. This was known as handover report which was a verbal communication of information. There were also various coloured notebooks, charts, patient care plans and doctors' notes. Nurses only left the ward for their entitled work breaks for lunch and coffee/tea time. Communication between nurses at this time became more informal if away from the ward, not only about personal issues but also about patients in their care.

Socialisation

The future of nursing culture as evident on this ward was dependent on transferring knowledge and skills related to caring for patients who had undergone surgical intervention.

This transfer was dependent on the student nurses who arrived on the ward at different periods of time during the year and also for certain lengths of time, being taught by qualified nurses who were more permanent members of the ward and were often called after the type of ward it was, e.g. surgical nurses. This allocation of student nurses to this ward and others like it was dependent on external forces that governed their whole initiation into nursing culture and also their socialisation into different ward areas. Student nurses are in fact a transient group but also nomadic over a period of time, in this case three years. They were seen as 'passing through' the ward culture (see Chapter 6).

Rituals

Based on the observations and interviews I undertook over a period of time as a researcher on the ward, I concluded that there were indeed rituals as related to the definition given by Turner (1969) and which were very clearly linked to time or temporality. The handover report and 'putting on uniforms' were two. Temporality was visible throughout the study, in the way nurses cared for patients, the way in which the hospital organisation influenced their work. Sacred and profane activities were central to their work as nurses, doing good and avoiding harm appeared central to their philosophy or work as nurses (see Chapters 4 and 5).

When we consider all these aspects of a nursing culture it is evident that they have been ongoing through time and that '*the process of becoming a nurse is both a social one*' (White & Ewan 1991) and an experiential one, where learning from their 'elders', or those qualified as nurses, is a critical part. White and Ewan (1991) believed that this needed to be differentiated from the process of earning a degree or qualification, and that in fact:

That latter process signifies that the individual has the required attitudes, skills and knowledge to practice competently. In contrast professional socialisation is the process by which the individual learns the culture of nursing: that combination of symbols, custom and shared meaning which makes nursing distinctive (p. 189).

Imagine this distinctiveness against other groups in any society or professions and how, without being told by anyone, through a number of symbols, carrying out certain activities and with a shared meaning, on seeing individuals in books, on television or film, or in a health care environment, their distinct appearance, the situation or backdrop to where they inhabit will immediately symbolise that they are a nurse.

Virginia Henderson (1978, p. 22) asking the question, is there a universal concept of nursing?, concluded that despite what nurses themselves and even doctors at that time might have thought the meaning and title should be, in some of Funk & Wagnalls' (1977) dictionary definitions she found: '*a female servant who takes care of young children*' or '*a person who cares for the sick, wounded or enfeebled, especially one who makes a profession of it*' which represented a public opinion that had to be taken into account.

I mention specifically these two definitions here in relation to public image in the early 1970s, as Henderson stated that (according to data from the International Labour Office 1976 and National Commission for the Study of Nursing Education 1970) this was '*still influenced by the fact that most nurses are women, the majority are not well educated, are not from the most privileged social class and are not well paid*'. Interestingly she cites the work of the anthropologist Margaret Mead (1949) in her analysis of 'male and female' in society, where '*the public concept of women's work is that it is "easy" compared with men*' and therefore this is reflected in how any women's work is viewed both socially and financially. Unfortunately, despite many changes in nursing as a profession and educationally, can we say without doubt that this long-lasting image of the nurse and nursing and indeed men and medicine does not still remain as part of the cultural image of nursing today? We will look closer at some of these issues of image and gender in later chapters.

Conclusion

This chapter has offered an introduction to nursing as a culture, especially as to how that has developed over time in certain countries, yet retained the essential characteristics that determine what nursing as both practice and occupation entails.

A cultural lens enables us to explore meaning to nursing and those that make up nursing groups. This lens indicates that, as in many 'tribal societies', although there are distinct or exclusive aspects to some nursing groups, as a collective the culture of all of them revolves around what is still called nursing, and that members of these groups are called nurses. This cultural lens will be used to explore some of these distinctive aspects of nursing and nurses in the other chapters.

References

Abel-Smith B (1960) *History of the Nursing Profession*, Heinemann Educational Publishers, London.

Allan H (2016) Becoming a patient. In H Allan, M Traynor, D Kelly & Smith, P, *Understanding Sociology in Nursing*, Sage, London.

Allen D (2001) *The Changing Shape of Nursing Practice: The Role of Nurses in the Hospital Division of Labour*, Routledge, London.

Allen D A (1997) The nursing-medical boundary: A negotiated order? *Sociology of Health and Illness*, 19 (4), 498–520.

Allen (2007) What do you do at work? Professional building and doing nursing, *International Nursing Review*, 54, 41–48.

Ashley J A (1976). *Hospitals, Paternalism, and the Role of the Nurse*, Teachers College Press, New York.

Beals R L, Hoijer H & Beals A R (1977) *An Introduction to Anthropology*, Macmillan, New York.

Davies C (1995) *Gender and the Professional Predicament in Nursing*, Open University Press, Buckingham.

Dorcy K S (1962) Built space and the socialization of nursing students, *Western Journal of Nursing Research*, 14(5), 632–644.

Equal Franchise Act (1928) UK Parliament, London (https://www.parliament.uk/about/living-heritage/transformingsociety/electionsvoting/womenvote/case-study-the-right-to-vote/the-right-to-vote/birmingham-and-the-equal-franchise/1928-equal-franchise-act/, accessed 7 May 2019).

Friedson E (1986) *Doctoring Together: A Study of Professional Social Control*, University of Chicago Press, Chicago.

Funk IK & Wagnalls (1977) Definitions from the *New Comprehensive International Dictionary of the English Language*. Encyclopedia Edition, Guild Press, New York. In V Henderson (1978) The concept of nursing, *Journal of Advanced Nursing*, 3(2), 113–130.

George S M (2005) *When Women Come First: Gender and Class in Transnational Migration*, University of California Press, Berkeley.

Goffman E (1961) *Asylums: Essays on the Social Situation of Mental Health Patients and other Inmates*, Penguin Books, Harmondsworth.

Gordon S (2005) *Nursing Against the Odds*, Cornell University Press, New York.

Gourlay J (2004) *Florence Nightingale and the Health of the Raj*, Routledge, Oxford.

Hector W (1973) *Mrs Bedford Fenwick: The Work of Mrs Bedford Fenwick and the Rise of Professional Nursing*, Royal College of Nursing and National Council of Nurses of the United Kingdom, London.

Helman C (2007) *Culture, Health and Illness*, 5th Edition, Hodder Arnold, London.

Helmstader C (2007) Florence Nightingale's opposition to state registration of nurses, *Nursing History Review*, 15, 155–165.

Henderson A (1994) Power and knowledge in nursing practice: The contribution of Foucault, *Journal of Advanced Nursing*, 20(5), 935–939.

Henderson V (1978) The concept of nursing, *Journal of Advanced Nursing*, 3(2), 113–130.

Holland C K (1993) An ethnographic study of nursing culture as an exploration for determining the existence of a system of ritual, *Journal of Advanced Nursing*, 18, 1461–1470.

Hugman R (1991) *Power in Caring Professions*, Macmillan, Basingstoke.

Johnson S E (2011) *A 'Suitable Role': Professional Identity and Nursing in India*, Unpublished PhD study, London School of Hygiene and Tropical Medicine, London (https://researchonline.lshtm.ac.uk/834552/1/550402.pdf, accessed 6 May 2019).

Kaminski J (2006) *Nursing through the lens of culture: A multiple gaze*, Unpublished study, University of British Columbia.

Lawler J (1991) *Behind the screens: Nursing, Somology and the Problem of the Body*, Churchill Livingstone, Edinburgh.

Lawton D (1989) *Education, Culture and the National Curriculum*, Hodder & Stoughton, London.

Littlewood J (1991) Care and ambiguity: Towards a concept of nursing. In P Holden & J Littlewood (1991) *Anthropology and Nursing*, Chapter 10, 170–189, Routledge, London.

MacGuire G (1968) The functioning of the 'set' in hospital controlled schemes of nurse training, *British Journal of Sociology*, 19(3), 271–283.

Mallidou AA, Cummings GG, Estabrooks CA & Giovannetti PB (2011) Nurse specialty subcultures and patient outcomes in acute care hospitals: A multiple-group structural equation modeling, *International Journal of Nursing Studies*, 48(1), 81–93.

Mead M (1949) *Male and Female*, Penguin Books, Harmondsworth.

Melosh B (1982) *The Physicians Hand: Work Culture and Conflict in American Nursing*, Temple University Press, Philadelphia.

Nair S (2012) *Moving with the Times: Gender, Status and Migration of Nurses in India*, Routledge, London.

Parsons T (1951) *The Social System*. Routledge & Kegan Paul, London.

United Kingdom Central Council for Nursing, Midwifery and Health Visiting (1986) *Project 2000: A New Preparation for Practice*, UKCC, London.

Rafferty A M (1996) *The Politics of Nursing Knowledge*, Routledge, London.

Reddy S (2015) *Nursing and Empire: Gendered Labor and Migration from India to the United States*, University of North Carolina Press, Chapel Hill.

Representation of the People Act (1918), UK parliament, London (https://www.parliament.uk/about/living-heritage/transformingsociety/electionsvoting/womenvote/case-study-the-right-to-vote/the-right-to-vote/birmingham-and-the-equal-franchise/1918-representation-of-the-people-act/).

Seymer L (1960) *Florence Nightingale's Nurses: The Nightingale Training School 1860 1960*, Pitman Medical, London.

Somjee G (1991) Social change in the nursing profession in India. In P Holden & J Littlewood (1991) *Anthropology and Nursing*, 31–55, Routledge, London.

Strouse S M & Nickerson C J (2016) Professional culture brokers: Nursing faculty perceptions of nursing culture and their role in student formation, *Nurse Education in Practice*, 18, 10–15.

Suominen T, Kovasim M & Ketola O (1997) Nursing culture – some viewpoints, *Journal of Advanced Nursing Studies*, 25, 186–190.

Svensson R (1996) The interplay between doctors and nurses – a negotiated order perspective, *Sociology of Health and Illness*, 18(3), 379–398.

Traynor M & Buus N (2016) Professional identity in nursing: UK students' explanations for poor standards of care. *Social Science & Medicine*, 166, 186–194.

Turner V (1969) *The Ritual Process: Structure and Anti-Structure*, Aladine De Gruyter, New York.

Volmer H M and Mills D L (1966) *Professionalisation*. Prentice-Hall, New Jersey.

White R & Ewan C E (1991) *Clinical Teaching in Nursing*, Chapman and Hall, London.

Wicks D (1998) *Nurses and Doctors at Work: Rethinking Professional Boundaries*, Open University Press, Buckingham.

Wilkins H (1993) Transcultural nursing: A selective review of the literature, 1985–1991, *Journal of Advanced Nursing*, 18(4) 602–612.

Wolf A, Ekman I & Dellenborg L (2012) Everyday practices at the medical ward: A 16-month ethnographic field study, *BMC Health Services Research*, 12(184).

Zerubavel E (1979) *Patterns of Time in Hospital Life: A Sociological Perspective*, University of Chicago Press, Chicago.

Further reading

1 Allan H, Traynor M, Kelly D & Smith P, *Understanding Sociology in Nursing*, Sage, London.

2 Allen D (2015) *The invisible work of nurses. Hospitals, organization and healthcare*. Routledge, London.

3 Hallet C (2010) *Celebrating Nurses – A Visual History*, FiL Rouge Press, London.

4 McDonald L (2018) *Florence Nightingale, Nursing and Health Care Today*. Springer Publishing Company, New York.

5 Nelson S & Gordon S (eds) (2006) *The Complexities of Care: Nursing Reconsidered*, ILR Press, Ithaca.

6 Nelson S & Rafferty A M (eds) (2010) *Notes on Nightingale: The Influence and Legacy of a Nursing Icon*, ILR Press, Ithaca.

7 Rafferty A M, Robinson J and Elkan R (1997) *Nursing History and the Politics of Welfare*, Routledge, London.

8 RobertsJ I and Group T M (1995) *Feminism and Nursing: An Historical Perspective on Power, Status and Political Activism in the Nursing Profession*, Praeger, Westport.

9 Wyatt L (2019) *The History of Nursing*, Amberley Publishing, Stroud.

3

RESEARCHING CULTURE

Principles of ethnography and ethnographic fieldwork

Karen Holland

Introduction

For anthropologists one of the important outcomes of their work is to make sure that what they seek to understand about any culture, or aspect of a culture, is made visible. This can be to enable them to deepen their own knowledge but also to enable others to gain an insight into various worlds through their descriptions of these. We saw in Chapter 1 the idea of the 'armchair anthropologist' where what was learnt was obtained from others' narratives or communications, such as Florence Nightingale in relation to public health issues in India. In her situation she did not go and see for herself, as it were, what the conditions and issues were in that country but relied on her exchange of letters and documentary evidence sent to her of what was possible or not.

However, those of you reading this book, and who have an interest in studying aspects of cultural life in different parts of the world or in your own country, will need some kind of framework to guide you to ensure that what you seek to make visible can be clearly seen or understood by others. For anthropologists the way of doing this is through using the principles of ethnographic inquiry in the first instance, followed by a written ethnography.

Ethnographic inquiry establishes the way in which a culture or part of a culture is explored, resulting in a description of what can be seen, or of the meanings of different actions and activities in an anthropological context. Geertz (1973) calls the 'focused picture' of what an ethnographer might write about a 'slice of culture', based on participant observation or interviews with individuals from what is called, in ethnographic terms, *'the field of study'*, whilst Clifford & Marcus (1986, p. 2) talk about writing ethnography and 'the making of texts'. Geertz notes the change in ethnographic accounts whereby *'a subgenre of ethnographic writing emerged, the self-reflexive fieldwork account'* (p. 14), which it appears in part is due to the publication of Malinowski's Mailu and Trobriand diaries (Malinowski 1967), which Clifford & Marcus (1986, p.14) claimed *'publicly upset the applecart'*. These diaries were published posthumously and had never been meant to become available as they were clearly in the style of what we now accept as self-reflection and our own analysis of ongoing fieldwork – that is of course beyond what are traditional fieldnotes.

This chapter will focus on the main methodology of research in studying cultures – through exploring ethnography, as both methodology and the written text, and how it has been used to research nursing and related health care contexts. The principles of ethnographic fieldwork, as well as the role of the researcher in gathering data and writing the ethnography, will be considered, alongside the newer approaches which link together ethnography with other views of the world. (See Further Reading for detailed texts on ethnography and its location in qualitative research methodologies, as well as examples of well-known written ethnographies.)

Ethnography

Ethnography has become a more common research methodology in nursing research (Mackenzie 1992; Holland 1993; Holland 1999; Williams 1989; Wolf 1986; Street 1992; Philpin 2004; Templeman 2015). However, ethnographic studies of nursing as a culture are not so visible. Before I discuss my exploration of different studies it is important that we are all starting from the same understanding of the principles of ethnography, especially as there is some dissonance as to what actually constitutes an ethnography. After reading many different textbooks, both on ethnography itself and those explaining qualitative research methodologies, it was clear that there were key similarities espoused by all of them; the main ones being that an ethnography is inextricably linked to anthropology and that it focuses on exploring culture or parts of a culture in order to make these visible and understood by others. Ethnography as a methodology belongs to the group of methodologies known as qualitative methodologies. According to Streubert & Carpenter (2011, p. 21):

> Qualitative researchers emphasize six significant characteristics in their research:
>
> 1 A belief in multiple realities
> 2 A commitment to identifying an approach to understanding that supports the phenomenon studied
> 3 A commitment to the participant's point of view
> 4 The conduct of inquiry in a way that limits disruption of the natural context of the phenomena of interest
> 5 Acknowledged participation of the researcher in the research process
> 6 The reporting of the data in a literary style rich with participant commentaries

Atkinson et al. (2007), in their handbook of ethnography, define it further than these six characteristics, whilst also acknowledging that there remain 'differences and tensions' due to a variety of perspectives. However, they do state that despite this, '*the ethnographic traditions do share many common features*' (p. 4). These common features include being

> 'grounded in a commitment to the first-hand experience and exploration of a particular social and cultural setting on the basis of (though not exclusively by) **participant observation. Observation** and **participation** … remain the characteristic features of the **ethnographic approach**. In many cases of course **fieldwork** entails the use of other research methods too. Participant observation alone would normally result in strange and unnatural behaviour were the observer not to talk with her or his hosts, so turning them into **informants or co-researchers**'. Hence **conversations** and

interviews are often indistinguishable from other forms of interactions and dialogue **in field research settings**. In literate societies the ethnographer may well draw on **textual materials as source of information** and **insight into how actors and institutions represent themselves and others** (p. 5) (my emphasis).

They indicate that from their own examination of the literature it would appear that:

> all too often authors and researchers are talking about the conduct of in-depth interviews – or focus groups – divorced from contexts of social actions or are amassing textual materials, diaries and biographies independently of the social contexts in which they are produced or used. These are often important ways of gaining principled understandings of social life and personal experience but should not necessarily be equated with ethnographic research (p. 5).

Ethnography as methodology is rooted in the discipline of anthropology, where the researcher is the essential means of obtaining an insight into the culture or aspects of the culture they are studying. It is, for the purpose of this book and chapter, taken for granted that, when discussing ethnographic studies, I will focus when possible on research that has encompassed anthropological principles, where it can be seen that some of these have been established as the theoretical and philosophical foundation to a study. I have highlighted in bold key words associated with ethnography as a methodology which is used by anthropological researchers. In addition I wish to also point out that just because some of these activities and actions are used by a researcher this does not necessarily mean that they are undertaking ethnography but simply using the methods associated with it, namely interviews and observation of different kinds, such as non-participant/participant observation and focus group interviews and individual interviews.

It is also important to note that you will find examples of differently named ethnography methodologies, reflecting either the type of fieldwork (urban ethnographies) or with an interdependent philosophy, such as feminist ethnography, autoethnography or critical ethnography.

The title of this chapter can be seen to include not only ethnography but ethnographic fieldwork or field research (Burgess 1982). This is because *the field* is where ethnographers conduct their research, that is '*researchers go to the location of the culture of interest*' (Streubert & Carpenter 2011, p. 172). Without gaining access to the field of study (used for both smaller focused aspects of a culture as well as a larger field) a researcher will not be able to conduct their ethnography. Autoethnography, however, does not of course adhere to these same boundaries (Muncey 2010).

In order to develop an understanding of what undertaking an ethnography can look like, this next section will look at major anthropological studies classed as ethnographies and their field of studies, followed by an exploration of nursing ethnographies as defined by the ethnographer/researcher.

Ethnographic studies: an insight into development of ethnography

One of the earliest British anthropologists was E B Tylor (1832–1917) who was instrumental in offering an initial definition of culture and who according to Kuper (1999, p. 56) stated that he had defined it in his book *Primitive Culture* as: '*Culture or Civilisation, **taken in its widest*** *ethnographic sense*, *is that complex whole, which includes knowledge, belief, art, morals, law, custom, and any other capabilities and habits acquired by man a member of society*' (Tylor 1871, cited in Kuper 1999).

Kuper (1999) noted that, considering Tylor's definition, in fact '*Culture is a whole; it is learned; and it includes practically everything you could think of, apart from biology*'. (See Chapters 1 and 2 for further discussion about culture and its definition.)

When considering these early anthropologists and their work it is important to remember as with any observation and reports of the time, that they were set against the Colonial developments that existed, explored in Chapter 1 when looking at the work of Florence Nightingale. You will see that the issue of ethnographers/anthropologists being used to promote Colonial policy is often noted in critiques of the development of anthropological studies (Hendry 2016). This issue of recognising the historical, social and political context in which an ethnographic study takes place is just as important today.

Tylor and others of that period did not undertake major fieldwork (in fact using the definition of an 'armchair anthropologist' seen in Chapter 1 we can see that this fitted Tylor's work and that of others like James George Frazer, author of *The Golden Bough* (Frazer 1993), concerning a study in magic and religion, and it wasn't until much later that we saw the rise of anthropological fieldwork that depended on the anthropologist being 'immersed' as it were in a specific cultural setting.

Bronislaw Malinowski, a Polish anthropologist, in his now 'classic' ethnography, *Argonauts of the Western Pacific*, based on his fieldwork with the Trobriand Islanders, is very clear in his view that to really explain what had been observed through living within any cultural group one should '*grasp the native's point of view, his relation to life, to realise his vision of his world*' (Malinowski 1922, p. 24). Burgess (1982) makes an important point, however, that Malinowski also '*considered that ethnographic material was only of value when it was possible to distinguish between direct observation, native statements and interpretations and the inferences of the author*', and that he also considered the inherent difficulties that could occur '*by the impact of the observer on the observed and the influence of the observer upon village life*' (p. 3).

These perspectives from Malinowski's work can be seen in the list of Streubert and Carpenter's reference to the characteristics of qualitative research and Atkinson et al.'s (2007) points about ethnography, previously discussed. I will examine some of these issues in discussing some of the nursing and related ethnographies in the next section.

We cannot discuss all the major anthropological studies that could be considered as background reading for conducting an ethnography in various 'cultural fields', so a list of some of these can be found in the Further Reading section along with a brief overview of their content. Some of the most well-known of these are: Evans-Pritchard's (1940) study of the Nuer in the Sudan, Evans-Pritchard's (1976) *Witchcraft, Oracles and Magic among the Azande* and Margaret Mead's (1928; 2001) *Coming of Age in Samoa*.

I would like to refer here to an important point that Margaret Mead set out in the preface to the 1973 edition of her book, that can in fact apply to many ethnographic accounts of the past where she says that:

> Some young critics have even asked me when am I going to revise this book and look unbelieving and angry when I say that to revise it would be impossible. It must remain, as all anthropological works must remain, exactly as it was written true to what I saw in Samoa and what I was able to convey of what I saw; true to the state of our knowledge

of human behaviour as it was in the mid 1920's; true to our hopes and fears for the future of the world (Mead 1973, p. xxiv).

When considering undertaking your own ethnographic study or undertaking a review of the ethnographic literature, it is important to remember that anything you read is of a specific time, and even though one researcher observed and wrote about one culture or cultural scene at a given period of time, another researcher might have arrived at a different point of view. This focuses of course on the actual 'doing of the ethnography' which then has to be transformed in the 'writing of the ethnography'.

Van Maanen (1988), in his book *Tales of the Field: On Writing Ethnography*, has an important viewpoint for readers of the **written ethnography** which I think is important to note here, when he states that:

> To produce an ethnography requires decisions about what to tell and how to tell it. These decisions are influenced by whom the writer plans to tell it to. Ethnographies are written with particular audiences in mind and reflect the presumptions carried by the authors regarding the attitudes, expectations and backgrounds of their intended readers (p. 25).

To explain this in the context of my research for this book I can illustrate with a personal example:

> I am Welsh and also speak Welsh. I was born in a small cottage hospital in a town in mid-Wales and lived until the age of 18 years of age in a very small Welsh village. During my Masters studies in medical social anthropology (later in my career) our course leader was Professor Ronnie (Ronald) Frankenberg, who brought anthropology to life in his teaching and his sharing his experiences with us of 'being in the field', not just in other countries but also 'at home' (Frankenberg 1957). The relationship between my background and his research is a 'sociological' study he undertook in a North Wales community (Pentrediwaith), where various descriptions of village life, especially those involving religious worship in different chapels/ churches resonated with my own growing up in the 1950s, where some of us went to the Methodist chapel, and some to the Church of England. His observations on the way villagers spoke Welsh then English in different circumstances was also acutely observed and would have also resonated with those from similar communities at the time it was published as well as it was for me today. Interestingly a colleague who had lived in Wales for some time, and of like mind to myself in relation to anthropology and ritual (the late Dr Sue Philpin), also related her experience of when and where those Welsh-speaking participants in an ICU where her research took place also did this (see Further Reading).

I was now reading his book or 'ethnography' as a 'different type of reader' to when it was published and it offered me a different kind of lens to what it must have been like living in that kind of village from his point of view.

The Introduction to the Frankenberg book is written by Max Gluckman (1957), himself a social anthropologist, and in his conclusion he makes a very important point related to the author's work – whereby: '*For a social anthropologist the interest in this book lies in its application of ideas developed in the study of tribal society to a community in Britain*'.

Although not a social anthropologist, this is where my interest is (and indeed for some of those colleagues we will consider in this book), in these wider areas of anthropological study that can be brought into the nursing research community, to enable us to offer another view of what we are, and what in fact we do as nurses in any society. We have a common history of where nursing as what we do now has stemmed from. Also from a wide variety of traditions that we have, regardless of our country of origin, we can identify with each other and what is at our core as a culture that recognises all this similarity and difference. One could argue that this is our inherited tradition and offers cultural patterns, much as in tribal societies narrated in the past and as now. The most important consideration, however, is that none are static, and that as in any society over time, nursing is in a continual state of change according to the context in which it exists.

So what ethnographies are available in nursing? I focused my search initially on views of nurse researchers in order to establish how ethnography as both methodology and methods, as well as a written ethnography in an anthropological tradition, was visible in the nursing literature. I considered full PhD studies and written ethnographies, articles in a wide range of journals as well as opinion or critical reviews of ethnography and its use and value in nursing. It would appear that there are minimal written ethnographies in nursing itself as in the traditional sense of those written by Frankenberg (1957) Richman (1983) Spradley (1970) and Spradley & Mann (1975) for example. However, there were some discovered in unpublished doctorate studies and articles accessed via the Internet. Before we consider some of these there is a need to determine further explanation of what an ethnography and ethnographic research entails.

Ethnography and nursing research

Aamodt (1982) drew on her own experiences of ethnographic research and teaching to offer a critical review of ethnography at that time. She offers an initial description of what it is considered to be, with a clear view that it can 'be both methodology and the written report for a research project' (p. 210) and that groups such as:

> first term students in a school of nursing, ... iron workers building a Denver skyscraper, represent sets of community members who share cultural rules for human activity in culturally specific scenes. Their story of their daily lives is ethnography (p. 201).

An interesting section of her paper focuses on the myths about ethnography, that 'were generated during many hours of discussion with anthropology and nursing colleagues' (p. 214). These were that:

1   All ethnography is alike.
2   Everyone can do ethnography.
3   Ethnography is easy.
4   All behavioural research questions demand ethnographic field methodologies.
5   Reliability and validity are of limited concern to ethnographers.
6   Findings based on intuitive responses in a field researcher are unimportant epistemologically.
7   Concepts/categories/variables can be transplanted from one cultural system to another and treated as if they are the same in both systems (p. 214).

She proceeded to unpack and in many ways debunk all these myths, using her own experiences (Aamodt 1981) and that of anthropologists such as Spradley (1979; 1980) and in her conclusions offered nurse ethnographers a goal whereby it '*is to continually seek out the meanings in the native's view in cultural and multicultural settings and search for ways of linking these understandings with concepts, processes and models for intervention in nursing care delivery systems*' (p. 220).

This goal remains an important one for nurses considering undertaking research which would enable an enhanced understanding of how patients in certain care situations, such as nursing homes for example, actually understand and exist in their cultural world. (See McLean 2007 in a study of nursing home care in the US for an ethnography of the person with dementia.)

This would also in turn enable health care professionals to further enhance the care that is received and also find new ways of working to support any change through undertaking research that also focuses on those who deliver the care itself.

This is a view supported by Savage (2000) who sees ethnography as being '*applied to health care issues in numerous ways*' (p. xxx), including the patients' views of their illness experience or how care is influenced by patients' cultural practices. She points out, too, that it can also be of value in understanding '*the organisation of health care*', in particular how it impacts on individuals and groups working in these organisations as well as the impact on the overall care delivery system that exists. Understanding how professional groups exist and develop in such organisational cultures is very important, for example when discussing the role of nurses or how student nurses learn to become nurses.

Brink & Edgecombe (2003) wrote a critique and a warning of what they called the phenomenon of the '*bastardisation of research designs*' (p. 1028) and the ways in which ethnography as a qualitative research design is being misused and misrepresented.

They point out that ethnography aims to be holistic and to try to describe what a people 'do' as well as what they 'believe'. They offer the explanation that '*Ethnography's signature is the study of naturally occurring human behaviour through observation*'.

This is of course a very simplistic explanation but they do also state that this signatory observation (participant) is used '*within a culturally and socially defined context*'.

Their focus is how researchers who are stating that they are '*doing or going to do participant observation*' or '*creating focus groups*' are not in fact doing ethnography. They are also quite vehement in a way when they state that '*some people believe that if they follow James* Spradley's (1979) *interviewing techniques as described in his book* The Ethnographic Interview, *they are doing ethnography*' (p. 1029). They make it clear that Spradley meant his books to be read and used in the context of anthropology students' understanding of ethnography. They contend that '*research studies, mislabelled as ethnography as appearing everywhere in the health care literature*' (p. 1030) and offer a series of questions as to why. They believe that if one changes too much of the core of the main methodology of research then it should then be changed and given a new name.

It is beyond the scope of this chapter to debate the premise of their beliefs but it is expected that readers will seek out the paper itself and discuss the questions they pose towards the end of their editorial. In terms of the basic premise of their argument, though, of calling something an ethnographic study when it isn't, there are published studies which state that they are adopting ethnographic approaches and not undertaking ethnography as defined by anthropologists and other researchers.

Now that we have considered what might not be an ethnography, we need to consider those that are clearly defined as such. I have chosen to call the next section 'making the familiar strange', as anyone undertaking an ethnography in their own field has to take into account the need to ensure that they undertake both an etic – 'stranger' (outsider) – view, as well as managing the emic (insider) view. This is one of the major challenges for ethnographers (Roberts 2007) and I believe that if nurses or nurse educators were not undertaking these various ethnographic studies into key aspects of their own specific nursing culture context then our understanding of our own cultural world would be very limited. There are few researchers who are from a nursing or health care background as it were who are undertaking nursing-specific ethnographies that are clearly immersed in anthropological concepts and theories.

Nursing ethnographies and 'making the familiar strange'

From searching the literature there appear to be some key areas of nursing culture where a number of ethnographic studies have been undertaken: examples being Intensive Care Units (ICU), mental health nursing (psychiatric nursing), nursing homes, rituals in nursing, the operating theatre, student nurses' clinical experiences and palliative care settings. Ethnographic studies of midwifery culture were also discovered and in particular the study by Hunt & Symonds (1995) on *The Social Meaning of Midwifery* in which the chapter on ethnography is also named 'treating the familiar as strange', and which is a recommended example of a written ethnography. A phrase that they use that resonated with me in relation to consideration of a nursing culture at large, as it were, is that: '*an ethnographic study must have a framework of historical and sociological explanation in order for it to be seen in full*' and also that: '*The purpose of ethnography is to show a familiar world from a different angle in order to make us question taken-for-granted assumptions and beliefs*' (p. 1).

Some of these ethnographies will be considered here and others can be found throughout the other chapters. Due to word space I can only focus on a few of these.

Unpublished doctorate studies

These were found in the main from the British Library ETHOS web site, which has proven an enormous and valuable resource during my research and education career. I have found a number of studies that are ethnographic in nature and offer a brief insight into some of them with the understanding that you as reader will both search for additional ethnographies not only from this important resource but also from other sites, but also read the ones I mention here in more depth.

1. The first ethnography is a thesis by Dr Anne Williams (1989) entitled *Interpreting an ethnography of nursing: Exploring boundaries of self, work and knowledge*. Her thesis is as much about her as an ethnographer as it is an ethnography. It makes for compelling reading and I will use her own words to explain the purpose of her thesis with regards to these two aspects of ethnographic research as she experienced them:

> Accounts of both ethnographic and nursing perspectives often tend to put forward one perspective or another in presenting a particular line of argument. My account departs from this approach insofar as I try to show how practices in both domains can be more

fully understood from a variety of overlapping perspectives. The boundaries I elucidate do not rigidly delineate the 'ethnographer' and 'the nurse', rather I try to demonstrate that there is a situational logic to how boundaries are drawn around experiences of self, work and knowledge by both myself and those I encounter in the field. That is to say, I explore how boundaries are continuously shifting, drawn and redrawn, interpreted and re-interpreted depending on a number of contextual features (Williams 1989, p i).

Personal note from Chapter Author

I can relate to some of her experience defined here when undertaking fieldwork (Holland 1999) observing student nurses in the field, sitting at the nurses' station in the middle of a very busy surgical ward. I was obviously, as Dr Williams herself, of the (nursing) culture as it were, and had learnt to separate myself from the field around me whilst simply noting down what was happening with the situation I was observing at the time, creating one boundary between myself and the nursing work being undertaken around me. However, for those I was observing and interviewing informally at key points during the day I was also a nurse teacher, creating another boundary as another self. This one, however, was much closer to the students than the boundary of me being a nurse in that particular field of study. The students were there on placement to learn to know what was required to underpin their care as well as to physically care for patients as part of their learning experience. This is where my three selves, as it were, came into being and the boundaries became very blurred as I had to stop my observations, make a note in my notebook and stop being a researcher – the reason being that a student and her mentor came to where I was sitting and immediately forgot I was there as a researcher, and started asking me to explain to them how a new piece of equipment to monitor blood glucose worked and how readings linked to diabetes! As this was important for the care of a patient I had to make an instant decision as a professional to switch from one self to another. *(Author reflecting on own experience in the field.)*

In retrospect and reading Williams's work today, for anyone with a nurse background undertaking ethnography those boundaries are very important when not only undertaking fieldwork but also when writing the ethnography itself. I would recommend anyone to access her work and read it in the context of being reflexive and how to value the importance of you as the researcher in the field that is also a part of it, in particular the fact that you explain the part 'I' (meaning you) played in both 'doing ethnography' and then describing the findings about what is the focus to the 'written ethnography'. In her case this was nursing itself.

2. The second ethnography to consider is very meaningful to my interest in ritual, but also the author was a colleague and friend and we were able to engage in meaningful discussion about this subject of interest where no explanation was required. Unfortunately Dr Philpin died in 2013 but I like to think that this work is her legacy to our understanding more about ethnography, nursing culture and rituals (see more in Chapter 5).

Her work focused on *An Interpretation of Ritual and Symbolism in an Intensive Therapy Unit* (Philpin 2004), where she explored its nursing culture and like my own research (Holland 1993) explored specific aspects of ritual and related symbolism. She undertook participant observation, interviews and documentary material that was found in the field. In terms of the ethnography as written, she makes clear that because of the way she '*has maintained a reflexive awareness of the various influences on the final written account*' the written ethnography aspects are discussed throughout the chapters as relevant.

Her major findings on rituals and symbolism I discuss in Chapter 5, the uniqueness of space and place in Chapter 4 and the issues around pollution and 'the body' in Chapter 8.

In relation, the place where she undertook her study also had an impact in the field as Dr Philpin was not only a nurse and researcher but she was also Welsh, that is her personal identity as being from Wales, where participants and others in the field of study also related to.

This background had an impact on the context of her study and the participants within it. This is an important aspect to consider when undertaking an ethnography where the 'place' (in this case a Welsh city) is as important as the actual field itself. She offers detailed explanations of how this other self of hers was reflected in the way in which participants described themselves and of course how they related to the patients and relatives in the ICU context. She calls that part of her study '*The role of the wider Welsh culture in Shaping Insider-Outsider Identity*' (p. 229).

This notion of personal identity in undertaking fieldwork such as this can also be seen in Johnson's (2010) PhD study, exploring '*professional identity and nursing in India*', where not only does she have her own personal identity as having Indian heritage but she was also researching the role that nurses have in a country where the status of nursing had not been considered professional like medicine. It was considered 'dirty work' (as seen by Somjee 1991) (see Chapter 8). Her methodology includes fieldwork, where, as with Philpin, her understanding of the local 'culture' helped her in developing relationships in the field.

One of the important issues that Philpin explains regarding the contribution her study made to nursing knowledge is that, in her words:

> I have demonstrated that using an anthropological approach, it is possible to tease out and make explicit the values inherent in nursing work. My methods of inquiry may be transposed to other areas of nursing work in order to discover latent meanings in nursing actions and their environment (p. 289).

I will be returning to her work in other chapters and I shall always remember our mutual backgrounds, as nurses, researchers 'doing ethnography' in nursing culture and rituals, and most importantly the fact we were both from the wider Welsh culture.

Published doctorate study

I am adding one study from the USA which had a major influence on my early experiences of both anthropology and ethnography. I was able to obtain the PhD of Zane Robinson Wolf (1986), entitled *Nursing Rituals in an Adult Acute Care Hospital: An Ethnography*, at the time of undertaking my own early foray into fieldwork (Holland 1993) and later purchased her published book based on this work: *Nurses' Work: The Sacred and the Profane* (Wolf 1988). Both are essential reading if undertaking ethnography of nursing culture. Her main research study is steeped in anthropology as well as sociology and nursing. She used the work of Turner (1969) and his study of rituals with the Ndembu tribe in Africa as well as Malinowski's (1954) work describing ritual within the context of magic, science and religion, and the rites of passage as discussed by Van Gennep (1960).

As well as using participant observation and interviewing for her study, Wolf also explored events and records '*such as patients' charts, staff meeting minutes and hospital forms*' (Wolf 1986, p. 24). She describes all her methods and experiences and then writes her ethnography around the five main findings along with a description of the settings and the people in the cultural scene she describes. Much of this latter description is not translated into her later publication of the PhD as a book, and both are discussed in greater depth in Chapter 5 focusing on rituals and nursing practice. The one aspect of Wolf's written doctorate that is unusual for an ethnography, is that she talks about herself in the research in the 'third person'.

For example:

> The investigator believes that her insider's knowledge of medical nursing units has resulted in increased sensitivity to the data present on the unit (p. 4).
>
> The investigator aimed to clarify the concept of nursing ritual, since this concept has not been explored extensively in the nursing literature (p. 6).
>
> The researcher used the ethnographic approach to provide detailed, descriptive data so that the investigation of nursing rituals could be embedded in the naturalistic context of an urban hospital's medical unit, 7H (p. 22).

I have concluded that this must have been due to an 'academic requirement' or possibly a similarity to early ethnographies which described what one saw as an observer rather than include the self in trying to make sense of what was observed. Her description of the 'cultural scenes' she observed are vivid (USA nursing and health care context) and as someone from the nursing culture in a very different health care system in the UK, they still resonated enough for me to understand what the nurses and patients were doing. In the preface to her book which stemmed from this exciting work, Wolf (1988) certainly included herself very clearly as part of her research.

The importance of Wolf's work is that it is a nursing ethnography that fits in with one of two definitions I have developed of what can be considered **nursing anthropology** (see p. 16 and Chapter 1: Definition 2), in her research of nursing rituals which she has clearly made visible through an anthropological lens, using the work, for example, of Victor Turner, Mary Mead and Arnold Van Gennep as well as others (Wolf 1988, p. ix):

> Nursing anthropology focuses on describing the nature of the nursing profession as a major cultural group that exists within various communities of practice in health care contexts. These communities exist as fields to be studied through an anthropological lens, encompassing the nurse as the main member of the culture whose focus of existence revolves around care work as nursing. This nursing work is set within various temporal, spatial and organisational contexts which are also rich fields for exploring the nature of this unique cultural group.

An important critical ethnographic study by Annette Street (1992) focuses on clinical nursing practice, which Giroux & McClaren (1992, p. 1) in their introduction state: '*is one of the first large-scale studies of medical knowledge and nursing culture undertaken by a critical social theorist working within the tradition of critical and feminist pedagogy.*'

In addition, and most importantly in relation to some of the chapters in this book, they also make the following claim about the study: '*in exploring the relationship between nursing knowledge and practice, it treats the production of meaning in its temporal, spatial, cultural and historical situatedness*' (p. 1).

We have already discussed the importance of the temporal, spatial and cultural aspects taken into consideration by Street (1992) who also adds the very important historical situation that has to be considered when examining the relationship between knowledge and practice as related to the culture of nursing. It is a very challenging and thought-provoking study which offers a different insight into aspects of nursing culture.

It is important that, after this brief insight into the use of ethnography in nursing practice, you access some of the other studies as per your own area of interest but mainly to consider how the ethnography itself was undertaken and written.

Undertaking an ethnographic study: an anthropological lens

In order for you to be able to read and critically review studies that are identified as ethnographies using an anthropological lens (Peacock 1986; 2001), it has been important in this chapter to briefly explore some of the essential elements that you would expect to identify in an ethnography. You will find that researchers have undertaken participant and non-participant observation, interviews, documentary analysis as well as engaging with key informants in the field. Specific reading is offered of texts that have been of value to myself in both undertaking ethnographic research as a novice and later in working with post-graduate students who wished to understand more about the possibility of undertaking an ethnographic study which would support an answer to their developing research questions. In undertaking ethnographic research as a novice I was especially influenced by John Van Maanen's (1988) work, *Tales of the Field*, as not only was I *'in pursuit of a culture'* (p. 13) but also trying to determine what I should do to make sure that others could see that what I had written about was understood. This book introduction stood out amongst many explanations:

> To write an ethnography requires at a minimum some understanding of the language, concepts, categories, practices, rules, beliefs and so forth, used by members of the written-about group. These are the stuff of culture, and they are what the fieldworker pursues. Such matters represent the ways of being and seeing for members of the culture examined and for the fieldworker as a student of that culture. The trick of ethnography is to adequately display the culture (or, more commonly, parts of the culture) in a way that is meaningful to the readers without great distortion (p. 13).

The chapters in this book are all written to offer different ways of thinking about nursing as a whole culture, including different aspects of nurses' work, nurses' education, nursing practice, nursing and patient care, organisations where nurses work. Anthropology offers a different lens to exploring meaning about what nursing is and what nurses do, and what can be made visible to others, that if they are from that cultural scene/field, for example, they are able to immediately resonate with it, as in Melia's (1987) words the researcher is *'telling it as it is'*. Any ethnography as research and as writing has to be seen in a specific cultural context, but also as Street (1992) very clearly indicated there is an importance attached to the temporal, spatial and the historical context in which that research is taking place.

Some studies I have read, however, do not specifically use the term ethnography nor ethnographic methods but they have had a long-lasting impact on the way we have come to understand social life and cultures in specific health and social care contexts. They also cross over disciplines such as sociology, psychology and anthropology; Erving Goffman's (1961) *Asylums* being one example and Julius Roth's (1963) *Timetables* being another. These examples can be found in the relevant chapters.

Conclusion

We have seen from this exploration of ethnography that if it is conducted using an anthropological lens that it can offer a valuable insight into the world of nurses and in turn a view that nursing as both profession and work can be considered a (nursing) culture.

Making this visible to others offers nurse researchers an invaluable opportunity to add to our understanding of the world that is 'nursing', and in particular its relationship to our initial raison d'être – that of caring for the sick – but also how we engage with those who are healthy in order to prevent them from getting ill. We can also begin to see the addition of evidence that could establish a specific field of its own, that of: Nursing Anthropology.

This exploration continues across all the other chapters.

References

Aamodt A A (1982) Examining ethnography for nurse researchers, *Western Journal of Nursing Research*, 4(2).

Atkinson P, Coffey A, Delemont S, Lofland J & Lofland L (2007) *Handbook of Ethnography*, Sage, London.

Brink P & Edgecombe N (2003) What is becoming of ethnography?, *Qualitative Health Research*, 13(7), 1028–1030.

Burgess R G (1982) *In the Field: An Introduction to Field Research*, Unwin Hyman, London.

Clifford J & Marcus G F (eds) (1986) *Writing Culture: The Poetics and Politics of Ethnography*, University of California Press, California.

Evans-Pritchard E E (1940) *The Nuer: A Description of the Modes of Livelihood and Political Institutions of a Nilotic People*. Oxford University Press, Oxford.

Evans-Pritchard E E (1976) *Witchcraft, Oracles and Magic among the Azande*. Clarendon Press, Oxford.

Frankenberg R (1957) *Village on the Border: A Social Study of Religion, Politics and Football in a North Wales Community*, Cohen & West, London.

Frazer J G (1993) *The Golden Bough Wordsworth Reference*, Wordsworth Edition, Ware.

Geertz C (1973) *Interpretation of Cultures*, Basic Books, New York.

Giroux H A & McClaren P L (1992) Introduction. In A F Street, *Inside Nursing – A Critical Ethnography of Clinical Nursing Practice*, State University of New York Press, New York.

Gluckman M (1957) Introduction. In R Frankenberg (1957) *Village on the Border: A Social Study of Religion, Politics and Football in a North Wales Community*, Cohen & West, London.

Goffman E (1961) *Asylums: Essays on the Social Situation of Mental Health Patients and other Inmates*, Penguin Books, Harmondsworth.

Hendry J (2016) *An Introduction to Social Anthropology*, 3rd Edition, Palgrave, London.

Holland C K (1993) An ethnographic study of nursing culture as an exploration for determining the existence of a system of ritual, *Journal of Advanced Nursing*, 18, 1461–1470.

Holland K (1999) A journey to becoming: The student nurse in transition, *Journal of Advanced Nursing*, 29(1), 1461–1470.

Hunt S & Symonds A (1995) *The Social Meaning of Midwifery*, Macmillan Press, Basingstoke.

Johnson S J (2010) *A 'Suitable Role': Professional Identity and Nursing in India*, Unpublished PhD study, London School of Hygiene and Tropical Medicine, London (https://researchonline.lshtm.ac.uk/834552/1/550402.pdf, accessed 6 May 2019).

Kuper A (1999) *Culture: The Anthropologists' Account*. Harvard University Press, Cambridge Massachusetts.

Mackenzie A F (1992) Learning from experience in the community: An ethnographic study of district nurse students, *Journal of Advanced Nursing*, 17, 682–691.

Malinowski B (1922) *Argonauts of the Western Pacific*, Routledge & Kegan Paul, London. Published in 2014 in Routledge Classics, London.

Malinowski B (1954) *Magic, Science and Religion*, Doubleday Anchor Books, New York. Reprinted by Martino Publishing, Mansfield Centre, CT.

Malinowski B (1967) *A Diary in the Strict Sense of the Term*, Stanford University Press, Stanford. Reissued in 1989 by Stanford University Press.

McLean A (2007) *The Person in Dementia: A Study of Nursing Home Care in the US*, Broadview Press, Peterborough, Ontario.

Mead M (1928, 1973, 2001) *Coming of Age in Samoa*. Republished in 2001 by Harper Perennial, New York.

Melia K (1987) *Learning and Working: The Occupational Socialisation of Nurses*, Tavistock Publications, London.

Muncey T (2010) *Creating Autoethnographies*, Sage, London.

Peacock J L (1986) *The Anthropological Lens: Harsh Light, Soft Focus*. Cambridge University Press, Cambridge. 2nd Edition published in 2001 by Cambridge University Press.

Philpin S M (2004) *An Interpretation of Ritual and Symbolism in an Intensive Therapy Unit*, Unpublished PhD study, University of Wales Swansea, Swansea.

Richman J (1983) *Traffic Wardens: An Ethnography of Street Administration*. Manchester University Press, Manchester.

Roberts D (2007) Ethnography and staying in your own nest, *Nurse Researcher*, 14(3), 15–24.

Roth J A (1963) *Timetables: Structuring the Passage of Time in Hospital Treatment and other Careers*, The Boobs-Merrill Company, Indianapolis.

Savage J (2000) Participative observation: Standing in the shoes of others?, *Qualitative Health Research*, 10 (3), 324–339.

Somjee G (1991) Social change in the nursing profession in India. In P Holden & J Littlewood (1991) *Anthropology and Nursing*, 31–55, Routledge, London.

Spradley J P (1970) *You Owe Yourself a Drunk: An Ethnography of Urban Nomads*, Little, Brown & Company, Boston.

Spradley J P (1979) *The Ethnographic Interview*, Holt, Rinehart and Winston, New York.

Spradley J P (1980) *Participant Observation*, Holt, Rinehart and Winston, New York.

Spradley J P & Mann B J (1975) *The Cocktail Waitress: Woman's Work in a Man's World*. John Wiley & Sons, New York.

Street A F (1992) *Inside Nursing – A Critical Ethnography of Clinical Nursing Practice*, State University of New York Press, New York.

Streubert H J & Carpenter D R (2011) *Qualitative Research in Nursing, Advancing the Humanistic Imperative*, Wolters Kluwer, Lippincott Williams & Wilkins, Philadelphia.

Templeman J (2015) *An ethnographic study of critical care nurses' experiences following the decision to withdraw life-sustaining treatment from patients in a UK intensive care unit*, Unpublished PhD study, University of Salford, Salford.

Turner V (1969) *The Ritual Process: Structure and Anti-Structure*, Aladine De Gruyter, New York.

Tylor E B (1871) *Primitive Culture*, London.

Van Gennep A (1960) *The Rites of Passage*, Routledge & Kegan Paul, London.

Van Maanen J (1988) *Tales of the Field: On Writing Ethnography*, 2nd Edition, University of Chicago Press, Chicago.

Williams A (1989) *Interpreting an ethnography of nursing: Exploring boundaries of self, work and knowledge*, Unpublished PhD study, University of Manchester, Manchester.

Wolf Z R (1986) *Nursing Rituals in an Adult Acute Care Hospital: An Ethnography*, Unpublished PhD study, University of Pennsylvania, Pennsylvania.

Wolf Z R (1988) *Nurses' Work: The Sacred and the Profane*, University of Pennsylvania, Pennsylvania.

Further reading

1 Coffey A (1999) *The Ethnographic Self: Fieldwork and the Representation of Identity*, Sage, London.
2 Coleman S & Collins P (2006) *Locating the Field – Space, Place and Context in Anthropology*, Berg, Oxford.

3 De Chesney M (ed.) *Nursing Research using Ethnography, Qualitative Designs and Methods in Nursing*, Springer Publishing Company, New York.
4 Germain C (1979) *The Cancer Unit – An Ethnography*, Nursing Resources, Massachusetts, USA.
5 Hammersley M (1998) *Reading Ethnographic Research*, 2nd Edition, Addison Wesley Longman, Harlow.
6 Jackson A (ed.) *Anthropology at Home* (1987) ASA Monograph 25, Tavistock Publications, London.
7 Roper J M & ShapiraJ (2000) *Ethnography in Nursing Research*, Sage Knowledge, London.
8 Street A (1995) *Nursing Replay: Researching Nursing Culture Together*. Churchill Livingstone, Edinburgh.

Ethnographies

9 Byerly E L (1970) *Registered Nurse Role Behaviour in the Hospital Sociocultural System: A Systems Approach* Unpublished PhD study, University of Washington, Washington.
10 Eschenbruch N (2007) *Nursing Stories. Life and Death in a German Hospice*, Berghahn Books, New York & Oxford.
11 Fish R (2018) *A Feminist Ethnography of Secure Wards for Women with Learning Disabilities*, Routledge, London.
12 Germain C *The Cancer Unit: An Ethnography*, Nursing Resources, Wakefield, USA.
13 Johnson K (1998) *Deinstitutionalising Women: An Ethnographic Study of Institutional Closure*, Cambridge University Press, Cambridge.
14 Johnson M (1997) *Nursing Power and Social Judgement*, Ashgate Publishing, Aldershot.
15 Johnson S E, Green J & Maben J (2014) A suitable job?: A qualitative study of becoming a nurse in the context of a globalising profession in India, *International Journal of Nursing Studies*, 51, 734–743.
16 Savage J (1995) *Nursing Intimacy: An Ethnographic Approach to Nurse-Patient Interaction*, Scutari Press, London.
17 Turner V W (1968) *The Drums of Affliction: A Study of Religious Processes among the Ndembu of Zambia*, International African Institute in Association with Hutchinson University Library for Africa, Hutchinson & Co., London.
18 Young M W (ed) *The Ethnography of Malinowski: The Trobriand Islands 1915–18*, Routledge & Kegan Paul, London.

4

TIME AND SPACE IN THE CONTEXT OF NURSING WORK

Karen Holland

Introduction

The interest in these two concepts began when I undertook fieldwork, firstly as a novice ethnographer searching for the existence of rituals in nursing culture, and later in my research focused on the transition of student nurses to becoming a qualified nurse.

I noted (Holland 1993) that time was an essential part of the daily lives of nurses on the surgical ward, including such activities as 'reporting (handover) time', and also the temporal structure of the whole day which remained the same in principle since Florence Nightingale's experience at Kaiserworth (Bullough & Bullough 1964). Later I was to see these same patterns emerge when observing student nurses in their clinical learning experiences (known as placements) which were in fact clearly delineated into set periods of time over a three-year programme of study to becoming a qualified nurse (Holland 1999).

Space, however, was a very elusive concept for me during both these observation periods although I had noted that there were very specific 'spaces' in the surgical ward where certain activities took place. Special space was also created by nurses for example when a patient died on the ward, seen when nurses closed the curtains around a patient's bed, creating a private space in the public and open place of the main ward.

During later research I was undertaking, I came across the work of Peter Gray (2004) in his doctorate study on spatiality and the lives of student nurses, and although his methodology was based in phenomenology, one of his main areas of interest to me was the experience of students in placements.

Given these links to student nurses' learning experiences to becoming a nurse and therefore learning to undertake nursing work for the future, I shall focus this chapter in part on the student nurse experience as regards time and space, whilst in Chapters 6 and 7, the issue of both time and space will also be explored in very different ways: one in relation to the student nurse socialisation and transition experiences, and the other in relation to nursing work in nursing culture, focusing on nursing in relation to the actual nature of nursing work in relation to patient care situations and how nursing work is seen in different cultural situations.

Nursing work

In order to establish how time and space impact on the daily lives of nurses it is important to initially establish what we mean by nursing work. The purpose and form of this nursing work has long been an issue of debate, not just from a philosophical stance but also from a more policy-orientated occupational one. The nature of nursing work I have found is such an eclectic mixture of skills and knowledge that it is impossible to describe it in a simplistic way, although many theorists such as Virginia Henderson (1960) have tried to define it.

Henderson's definitions are the most established and remain for many the most important in the history of nursing in trying to capture what nurses did in their work and this was seen through her actual belief of the function of a nurse. The overarching definitions were underpinned by further explanations of major concepts and sub-concepts that were unpacked in relation to the overarching definitions. These are:

> I believe that the function the nurse performs is primarily an independent one – that of acting for the patient when he lacks knowledge, physical strength, or the will to act for himself as he would ordinarily act in health, or in carrying out prescribed therapy. This function is seen as complex and creative, as offering unlimited opportunity for the application of the physical, biological, and social sciences and the development of skills based on them (Henderson 1960).
>
> the unique function of the nurse is to assist the individual, sick or well, in the performance of those activities contributing to health or its recovery (or to a peaceful death) that he would perform unaided if he had the necessary strength, will or knowledge. And to do this in such a way as to help him gain independence as rapidly as possible (Henderson 1991).

There are other definitions such as those from the International Council of Nurses (see: http://www.icn.ch/who-we-are/icn-definition-of-nursing/) and the World Health Organisation (see: http://www.who.int/topics/nursing/en/) but the basic principles of these are based on Virginia Henderson's early work. In the UK, the Royal College of Nursing produced an important paper called *Defining Nursing* (RCN 2014) explaining why it was now very important that the work of nursing be clarified and offering a range of six characteristics of nursing which they then explored. One statement stood out for me and resonated with my own beliefs concerning the uniqueness of nursing:

> The definition of nursing that is presented in this document is expressed in the form of a core explanation supported by six defining characteristics …. **It is important to recognise that nursing is the totality: while some parts of the definition are shared with other health care professions, the uniqueness of nursing lies in their combination**. The definition takes account of the great diversity of nursing, which includes the care of people who are healthy as well as those who are sick, and of groups of people as well as individuals. The definition expresses the common core of nursing which remains constant (RCN 2014, p. 3) (my emphasis).

Like all work, nursing can be broken down into distinct tasks or skills but what makes nursing work different is that those who are qualified to do so can use their skills in such a way that they integrate it into a different context every time they meet a different patient. Nursing work in that sense is unique, in that each nurse–patient relationship is unique (not in form but possibly content); each encounter bringing with it a need to undertake nursing work in an individualised way. Given that nursing is this 'unique blend' as it were, I liken it to a kaleidoscope – unique at each turn of a nurse–patient interaction and set within a different temporal, spatial but also cultural context. The student nurse is required to gain practice of such relationships within such context – each experience being a separate, bounded 'time specified' experience according to the prescriptive directive of a curriculum that directs their journey and initiation into the world of nursing work (see Chapter 6). Nursing work in relation to labour is explored in Chapter 7.

Time and space in the culture of nursing work

For any student wishing to learn to become a nurse there is a professional requirement that this experience is guided by explicit 'rules' prescribed as to what is to be included in a curriculum by the Nursing and Midwifery Council (NMC) in the UK and similar professional bodies in other countries. In the UK as in other European countries presently this is also overlaid with other EU laws, and important for this chapter is the number of hours that students have to experience in clinical placements. This amounts to 50% of their three-year or equivalent programme of study in a university, working in partnership with organisations where the student will get to engage in both learning about nursing work and what it entails but also how to engage in this nursing work. This is broken down into specific time of 2,300 hours of theory and 2,300 hours of practice: 4,600 hours in total. The specific detail of how these hours are defined further can be seen in the progression of the student nurse through their learning journey to become registered (qualified) nurses. The hours are further defined into 'blocks' of time periods called placements, which have the uniqueness of being (in the main) parallel with those 'illness' experiences of the patient. They are what one can call 'bounded' experiences, given the specific time and space the student will be allocated in order to achieve what they need to make the transition to becoming a qualified nurse. (We explore this in more detail in Chapter 6.)

However, given the importance of the relationship between the student nurse and the patient in such spaces, we need to understand more about nursing work and how these spaces are seen and/or established.

Grint (2005, p. 6) explains that '*work is intimately related to the temporal, spatial and cultural conditions in existence*' but before we explore these concepts further we need to explore why this 'nursing work' is required in the first instance.

Nursing work exists because of the vulnerability of society to ill health with its consequent impact on both the individual who succumbs to illness and their immediate others. Illness, however, disturbs the balance of social living and societies find different ways of containing its potential impact. It is for this reason that we saw the building of hospitals and the subsequent removal of certain sick people from the home to the hospital. For Littlewood (1991, p. 178):

> The sick person has transgressed social rules, has disobeyed accepted ideas on behaviour in space and time. He is separated off, contained, or isolated in order not to contaminate others. His ideas of time and space are disturbed and he needs to go through a cleansing

and healing process in order to be made well. For this process to occur, he is traditionally removed to the hospital – removed from his home and his culture – and is subjected to being undressed, given a bath or enema and placed in a space identical in most respects to that of other sick people on the ward.

It has to be noted here that how this 'hospitalisation' experience happens has changed since 1991, especially when not every patient who is diagnosed as 'sick' is removed from their home, but in principle the notion of separation from home and the norm as in away from 'well people' remains. I will illustrate this by offering two personal experiences.

Personal experience of time and space to illustrate meaning: as a Realist Tale (Van Maanen 1988)

Two personal experiences in 2016 illustrated the difference to how this transgression and notion of 'being sick' happens. In brief, **my first experience** was a planned admission to hospital to have a replacement knee operation. Certainly the undressing part, leaving behind my normal self, took place as did the pre-operative preparation or ritual cleansing experienced by the majority of patients undergoing surgery. Time as I normally experienced it through looking at a watch or clock became meaningless as my watch was removed and my relationship to time now related to how I counted my fellow patients going to the operating theatre in the order of where I fitted in on the surgeon's 'listed' surgery times. I stayed in hospital, in my own bed space, for 2 days, which I thought incredible when I reflected on my own experience of caring for people during my own training in the late 1960s, when patients who had similar surgery to mine were in hospital for up to three whole weeks! This change in specific times in hospital according to a specific surgical procedure is where the development of medicine and nursing has had a major impact on timelines related to illness. Not only this but it also impacted on the health and well-being of the patient as I was able to leave that hospital environment and go home. I did not feel despite the major surgery that I was in fact suffering from an illness. In addition, my being 'released' from the hospital was not the end of being confined in one space, as in my own home I had to create another space which more or less mirrored that of the hospital bed and a small ward. The daily routine continued as before, with medication times, exercise time, sleep time and of course family visiting time.

My second experience, however, was completely different in terms of both time and space. It also had a much more profound impact on my health and well-being. A brief insider view only is possible here. I was taken to the hospital in an emergency ambulance to the accident and emergency (A&E) department, a very different space to a hospital ward, and where the private and public aspects of illness clashed in a very unique way. Here the priority was focused on ensuring that patients such as myself were given a rapid diagnosis and life-saving treatment. I was transferred from the space inside the ambulance to the new space of the A&E Department, to occupy a space in a corridor until what could be called a 'diagnostic' space was available. The space I then occupied was a trolley surrounded by curtains which were left opened at the front to allow the nursing and medical team access to observe me, and were only closed when they either needed to undertake some kind of treatment or I needed to use the commode. I had plenty of time (without knowing what the actual clock time was.) following the emergency care I was given, to observe what was happening around me and I thought (when I felt recovered from the initial concerns of the doctors) of the wonderful opportunity to undertake non-participant observation. However, my sense of self and others around me whilst lying on the trolley and in that space took on new meaning, as we were now part of the waiting time directive governing the times that patients stay in A&E departments. Three hours waiting for a ward bed was well within this time frame.

Once stabilised I then experienced removal to a ward again but this time in a different space (named as a medical ward which had been allocated an initial and a number) and in addition I had the experience of being closely watched again by the nurses as my initial bed was opposite the nurses' ward station. The panopticon experience lived!

I was kept away from my home in hospital for four whole days (in themselves part of the bigger pattern of Time), where the space I occupied consisted of a bed in a small four-bedded unit as part of the bigger space of the ward. Time, in terms of moving from morning to afternoon to evening and then night, now became focused on different kinds of time, such as medicine time, lunch time, lights-out time, visiting time (when 'outsiders' were allowed in to visit patients). All these were part of the overall daily routine activities managed by nurses and other health care workers. During those four days, time as I normally experienced it at home, such as waking up, taking tablets, getting up, now lost meaning as I developed an awareness of myself where my normal concept of time and activities were no longer relevant. This can be disorientating, but from an insider view of being a nurse it was less so for me but was clearly an alien world for others. The ebb and flow of patterns of activities and people now became the focus of my day. Watching the student nurses, watching the patients come and go from the ward, waiting for my family to visit, hoping for time to sleep. The space I occupied from which to observe all this remained the hospital bed, and the only other space I was allowed to occupy was that of the nearby bathroom as required. Even here, however, I was not allowed total personal space as my illness required further observation.

These two examples of my experience are taking place every day somewhere around the world, albeit in different cultural contexts but also in different time zones that are defined for us. Littlewood's (1991) view of the hospital where I was also 'allowed to be sick' (as a personal experience) became very much a reality.

The hospital: time and space

Student nurses, in their learning to become nurses, are required to experience these kinds of hospital spaces (as those I encountered) as well as similar others where the patient who is diagnosed as sick can actually stay in their own home or be removed to a different kind of space, such as a hospice. One is clearly a public space of a hospital and the other a private social space of the patient's own home. A hospice, it could be argued, offers a sense of both.

Strauss et al. (1963) likened a hospital to a workplace and stated that:

> a hospital consists of variegated workshops ... places where different kinds of work are going on, where very different resources (space, skills, rates of labour force, equipment, drugs, supplies and the like) are required to carry out their work, where divisions of labour are amazingly different, though all this is in direct or indirect service of managing patients' illnesses.

The hospital, however, is according to Zerubavel (1979a, p. xix) 'one of the few organisations or facilities, whose operation around the clock, seven days a week and 365 days a year, dictated primarily *by its moral "raison d'être", rather than by consideration of productivity and profit'*. He points out that *'in almost every culture known to us, health and illness are symbolically located in the sacred domain, and that makes the hospital an example of a formal organisation which is governed by practical, as well as moral, principles'* (p. xviii).

The time that patients may spend in hospital, plus the way in which that time is organised and managed, also has an influence on both the student experience of nursing work and that of the qualified nurse who is tasked with ensuring that the student learns the skills and knowledge required for caring for patients (see Chapter 6).

Time and space are, according to Helman (1992, p. 36), *'among the core building blocks of any culture'* and states that *'there are differences in the notion of time between societies and between different populations within these societies'*. In particular he focuses on the two forms of time as defined by Hall (1984), namely monochromic and polychronic.

Monochronic time is governed by linearity *'as a line or ribbon stretching from past to future and divided into compartments or segments, such as years, hours, minutes or seconds'*. It is also, in its uniqueness, as originating outside the individual *'a form of external order imposed on the chaotic lives of humanity'*.

Polychronic time as proposed by Hall (1984), however, *'involves doing many things at once, and which stresses involvement of people and completion of transactions, rather than adherence to preset schedules'* (Helman 1992: 38). Individuals who exist in polychronic time *'are orientated towards people, human relationships and the family, which is the core of their existence'*.

If we apply these concepts to nursing work, it could be argued that nursing by its very human relationship-focused nature is polychronic, yet it exists as a job within mainly monochronic organisations. Jones (2001) supports this notion that nursing in the UK at least, because of the way in which clock and calendar time govern nursing activities and professional training, *'... exists within the framework of the linear monochronic model'* (p. 152).

Time, nursing work and culture

Given that nursing also exists in a cultural context and that different cultures may have their own view of time, this could have a significant impact on the way in which nursing work is undertaken. Giger & Davidhizar (2008) for example cite many instances of the impact of time on nursing care and work practices. They note that: *'when people of different cultures interact, as is frequently the case in health care settings, there is a great potential for misunderstanding'* (p. 119).

Their particular transcultural nursing model supports the view that *'transcultural nursing is viewed as a culturally competent field that is client centred and research focused'* (Giger & Davidhizar 2008, p. 5), and most importantly when it comes to the focus of this chapter, they have developed a framework for nurses to use which encompasses both time and space in relation to delivery of culturally appropriate care. As discussed in Chapter 2, whatever views one has of transcultural nursing and the drive for nurses to be culturally competent across many cultures, it is important for nurses to have an awareness of cultural differences in the way time is both lived and experienced. Their book offers a broad introduction to the model and these two important concepts but also offers an insight, through what some may deem a 'recipe book approach', to how various cultural groups in the USA perceive and experience time and space as part of the whole model, including how it impacts on nursing practice. I learnt, for example, that scheduling appointments for health care in the Yup'ik and Inupiat peoples of Alaska is a challenge because of the way present time is perceived, and that many patients preferred to come to the clinic when they felt like it (Giger & Davidhizar 2008, p. 337).

Their life inside the Arctic Circle also has a major impact on the wider aspect of time as measured by length of day time and night time. We can I think learn much from their experiences when we consider the issue of shift patterns in nursing work.

We know that nursing work takes place in both hospital and non-hospital environments, and that time governs what nurses do at specific times of the day and night. In my exploration of nursing ritual in a hospital ward (Holland 1993) the nurses were part of the workforce of the hospital and as such were subject to a working day in which social and clock time as defined by Zerubavel (1981) was identified.

They had organised rotas for when they were at work that fitted the overall organisational pattern of work in a hospital. Work activities governed by time (for example four-hourly – physiological-related – observations) were clearly defined; all revolving around the patients.

This temporal structure in which nursing work takes place was present even in Kaiserworth (Bullough & Bullough 1964, p. 85), which Florence Nightingale first visited in 1850 (Smith 1972):

> Nurses at Kaiserworth wore blue print gowns and white caps. Their workday was long and hard. They rose at 5am, made beds, swept their rooms, and then went to the wards to help with the patients before breakfast. Around 6.15am they had a light breakfast perhaps a cup of coffee, and then in line with their calling as deaconesses devoted some time to prayer. They then returned to the wards where they gave the patients their medicines and began washing and dressing the patients. At about 8 or 8.30am the physicians began their rounds accompanied on each ward by the ward supervisor. After this time there was usually a coffee break for both patients and nurses (Bullough & Bullough 1964, p. 85).

I had observed this type of pattern when undertaking fieldwork, as both clock time which governed the time the nurses started their working day and followed, as in Kaiserworth, with periods of social time where the nurses engaged in 'non-work' (Holland 1993, p. 1466). One kind of time period that stood out in the culture of the ward was that of 'reporting time' where it appeared a cultural rule, '*an unwritten law that all nurses should attend*', and I had concluded that '*it would appear to be a way of ensuring that social order is maintained within the group be enforcing cohesion and interaction*' (p. 1467).

In both situations the order of the day with regards to time was and still is built around the organisational rules which existed in the hospital. In fact in the narrative of my own personal experience already seen, the imposition of specific time schedules was critical to ensuring not only smooth running of the operating theatre working time for the operating team, but was also influenced by an established time expectancy for each operation. There was an established 'normal time' for my knee replacement, for example, and on this rested the time it would then take for other patients to follow me for their surgery. The hospital and every aspect of its working is governed by the intricate and indeed interdependent temporal order, or as Zerubavel suggested calling it, in his concluding observations, the 'sociotemporal order' (Zerubavel 1979a, p. 105).

This is an important direction which helps understand that my individual time line for surgery cannot be seen in isolation from my co-patients that morning, nor indeed the impact of maintaining scheduling on the whole of the nurses' work on the ward and also those working in the operating theatre. Roth (1963) in his work on timetables noted that '*the time of surgery is important in the timetable because patients always have a definite conception of how long one has to remain in hospital after surgery'* (p. 6). His comment related to his timetable of the patient with TB (diagnosed Tuberculosis) but its relevance still influences the timetable attached to any patient undergoing surgery today. The work of the surgeon and the surgical team as well as the ward team is governed by scheduling. In relation to this Zerubavel (1979a:106) stated that:

> The structural components of the sociotemporal order are collectivities, and its major institutionalised representations – the schedule, the calendar and the timetable – are essentially of a collective nature. Schedules are usually shared by collective entities and are not designed for particular persons on an individual basis.

An example of a new nursing development which in my view was a casualty of this particular nature of schedules having to work for the collective nature rather than the individual when it came to individualised patient care, was that of primary nursing. This new way of delivering care was developed by Marie Manthey (1980) as a way to improve the way care was delivered to patients and her motivation defined as the *'re-humanisation of hospital care'* (p. xvii). The central concept for nurses was a *'decentralised decision making'* process which allowed a more personalised approach by nurses to care for smaller numbers of patients but also enabled the patient to experience a more individualised form of care, where their needs would become more important than that of the wider collective around them. Their Primary Nurse would be the main decision maker of their care. Scheduling of care work became focused on an individual basis, as did the need to individualise specific timetables such as medicine administration according to the patient's own needs.

In principle it was a model that attracted those managing hospital care at that time, and no doubt as the model was developed in the context of a US health care system, implementing some of its ideologies into the UK NHS system mitigated against its implementation in the way Manthey's philosophy was meant. The role of the *named nurse* was born out of this attempt to manage care differently. It is also another example where the culture of the NHS organisation itself at that time had an impact on care delivery.

Adhering to the main principle of the delivery of care according to the individual patient's needs, in a hospital governed by major scheduling as well as managing care, for example, to 30 individuals in one ward space, would have been a challenge in any health care context. From personal experience of its implementation one of the other major challenges focused on a time issue in relation to decision making, whereby there had to be *'a clear allocation of a 24 hours a day responsibility at the head nurse and middle management levels of a department to ensure that adequate continuity between shifts is successfully maintained'* (Manthey 1980, p. 68).

Of course, as with many other initiatives which were implemented in the UK but their origins had been developed in the USA where the culture of health care delivery and the nature of its implementation was very different, this new development of primary nursing, one could argue, became a casualty of an organisational culture where time, as both monochronic and polychronic, along with the kind of personnel levels to deliver wholesale individualised care as per primary nursing, eroded away its core focus and was transposed into a new term which could be both visible and accepted as another option in a changing health care scenario: that of the named nurse. This term was adopted in the UK instead of the Manthey one of primary nursing, explained in a mental health context by Shebini et al.

(2008) where in fact the patient-to-nurse ratio was very different, as was the nature of the space in which many patients at the time, with mental illness requiring hospitalisation, were actually cared for.

I am conscious that this extended explanation with regards to primary nursing and named nurse might appear an indulgence as an author, but for those who are not nurses reading this chapter it is essential that even a brief overview is necessary to illustrate how certain nursing work time allocation is impacted by the organisational culture in which patient care exists.

The implementation of primary nursing as a new way of care delivery was also influenced by the context in which the majority of it was planned to take place, that of the spatial context of the hospital. Consider the personal experiences described previously when considering how the concept of the named nurse could be realistically implemented in such care environments as the Emergency Department, both in terms of time and space.

Spatial contexts of nursing work

What is meant by space? In its simplest terms it means:

> A continuous area or expanse which is free, available, or unoccupied.
> The dimensions of height, depth, and width within which all things exist and move.
> (See English Oxford Living Dictionaries: https://en.oxforddictionaries.com/definition/space)

We have already seen how the first definition is visible in nursing contexts as a space that can be seen, such as a ward area, but in fact the second definition concerning the physical dimensions of height, depth and width, creating a very different spatial context which is not as tangible or visible other than in relation to other sets of dimensions – creating space in fact – is not as easy to imagine in relation to nursing work. One can imagine these three dimensions by considering how hand luggage space is defined – not as how much space is inside the luggage but of course its size outside. By definition this will in turn establish how much the inside space is from their required dimensions. However, as many of us know when carefully packing for a holiday, two suitcases of the same dimensions outside do not always translate to the same space inside!

One major area where this second definition is important is when a new hospital or clinic is being designed, as all outside measurements will create different kinds of inside space that are required to deliver care. Dorcy (1992) calls this 'built space' and considers how this impacts on the socialisation process of the student nurse. This is a unique paper reporting on what the author calls an 'historical-ethnographic study' focusing on Nursing School building from 1928 (p. 632). She stated that: *'Architecture is a silent reflection of cultural beliefs and values'* and that *'The role of architecture within the socialisation of nurses is an implicit dimension of the education of nurses'*.

Before we look at the way in which built space has influenced the world of the student nurse as explored by Dorcy (1992) and indeed nursing work generally, I would like to consider the work of Antonacopoulou (2002) in regards to learning and space.

Antonacopoulou (2002), in her examination of the relationship between space and learning, provides us with a possible framework for examining the relationship between where student nurses learn to undertake nursing work and their other learning, and she considered that the *'where and when of learning taking place are neglected aspects of organisation learning debates'* (p. 2).

She asks the question: what is space? and identifies the following dimensions of space from the literature, namely: space as an area of struggle; space as order and censorship; spaces as artefact and representation; space as action; space as multiplicity and specificity and: space as a journey. In her brief description of these dimensions she offers an insight into their potential value for us in exploring space in the context of nursing work.

Space as artefact and representation, for example, enables us to consider the learning spaces that the student nurse has to engage with in any placement. These are the bounded spaces already defined and linked to patients' medical journey and diagnosis, such as the orthopaedic ward for different surgical intervention in relation to the skeletal system such as repairing a fractured femur. Immediately this space represents an image, and is associated with specific artefacts related to this idea of 'orthopaedics' and fractured femurs. The student nurse has to learn to recognise a whole new language of symbols associated with this learning space, which is the workplace for qualified nurses, and in turn learn what everything in that space represents as part of the nursing culture on that ward. If you are a nurse reading this you will of course immediately associate your understanding through word association and images of what it involves. Some of you as non-nurses may refer to your own personal experience of a visit to a friend or family member in an 'orthopaedic' ward or possibly even your own insider experience.

In contrast, however, the learning space (for the student nurse) in a community setting and the patient's home is represented very differently because the focus is now 'domiciliary space'. Twigg (1999, p. 384), for example, notes that firstly *careworkers in entering the home come as guests – they have to be invited in; they then have to negotiate the "spatial ordering within the home"* which mirrors the public and private between home and the outside world; for example, the bathroom becomes a private space.

In previous field work I had concluded (Holland 1993) that there were social structures, as organised patterns of relations in place within the hospital. These were known as the surgical wards, *'created especially to house the sick in society'* (Littlewood 1991). Each ward was separated from others within the hospital building itself and the whole hospital had its own organisational culture. The patients in these wards were 'allowed into these spaces' on the basis that they had a medically diagnosed illness which had required surgical intervention.

One can view these wards, as a patient's home, or a health centre as bounded spaces, or what Savage (1995) calls symbolic space, both in terms of actual physical boundaries or individual walls within each and the overall building itself. Different spaces have different functions in terms of what nursing work takes place in them. For example, as I illustrated previously with my own experience, the accident and emergency department in a hospital is a very different physical space to that of an intensive care unit – both in terms of physical layout and where it is placed in a hospital.

How a ward is designed in terms of space, for example, has a major impact on nursing work and how it is carried out. A ward can also be considered a place in the hospital which Jowsey et al. (2012) refer to as *'defined areas within health service environments whilst the term "space" referred to often abstract meanings, boundaries and uses associated with places'* (p. 197).

Florence Nightingale (1863) considered there were essential elements of ward design to ensure efficiency, namely: the bringing together of things needed for nursing in the area of work, ease of supervision of patients and staff, distribution of the sick in convenient numbers for attendance and position of nursing rooms to ensure a full view of the ward both day and night. Littlewood (1991, p. 179) contends that:

Personal space on a hospital ward changes from minute to minute and is affected by population density (bed occupancy) purposes of approaches (injections, casual conversation), fixed locations (beds), character of social occasion (visiting time, ward rounds). The nurse may move the curtains around a bed to expand or contract the patient's personal space. The curtains, bed and its associated locker define the areas within which one functions.

Savage (1995: 89) in her study of nurse–patient interactions on a hospital ward found that nurses described the 'patient's space' in the same way, and that the boundaries of this space 'corresponded with where the curtains hung, whether or not these were pulled around the patient's bed'. Both Savage (1995) and Lawler (1991) found that the notion of patients' space was linked to the issue of privacy. Some of these spaces are also associated with potentially distressing nursing work, such as those found in a hospice, which is a large space built especially for those who are dying from a terminal illness. Hockey (1990, p. 166) describes these types of spaces as:

> Spanning the boundary between life and death, hospices represent spaces within which the experience and the idea of transition is demonstrated and made possible. Thus the boundary between the hospice and the surrounding community is the site of maximal movement, a public space where the life/death continuum is powerfully suggested.

Death can of course occur within the boundary of the hospital ward and managing this is often associated with what Wolf (1988) calls nursing rituals (see Chapters 5 and 10). Time and space can also come together in life or death situations, especially in critical situations involving a patient, and where normally conscious thought is not apparent. However, here is an example of what happened when a student nurse was asked to reflect on one experience (in an Accident and Emergency Department setting which is a place in a hospital: the background was the resuscitation room – a dedicated space for very seriously ill people – within the overall department. The scenario taking place was validated by the student's mentor in clinical placement and I had permission to use it in my research):

> Student AB63: *I was amazed at the depth of concentration I had upon the patient, watching his chest rise and fall with oxygen being pumped into his lungs by the team leader. I was hoping for some signs of life. My arms started to ache and I could feel the heat from the over bed light beginning to make me sweat and feel hot.* **I looked up to see the time. I had been doing compressions for nearly ten minutes. I thought of having a break**. *I looked around for someone to take over, there was nobody free. They were all busy carrying out their own tasks for the patient. I could carry on. I was not exhausted **but I felt all the time I needed a rest. I did wonder how long the team were going to keep on trying** and who out of the team it would be to disengage procedures …the **clock was now showing twenty past one, I had now been doing CPR for twenty minutes** (my emphasis).*

The patient here could also be seen, in Zerubavel's (1979b, p. 91) view, as being a 'temporal unit of work', in terms of measuring the passage of time. The student is clearly demonstrating a major focus on the patient, whereby time is measured in relation to the patient himself over a certain period (of time). It also offers through their intense focus on the patient, an image of the space where the procedure was taking place but also the very focused space in which this student was carrying out a procedure. Having an inside experience of such a scenario enabled me to interpret the scene that surrounded this focused example, especially the space (a bed in a resuscitation room in an A&E Department) where it took place and the forgetting about 'time' itself when a life-saving procedure was happening; whilst for the student they reported their experience as it was or, as Melia states, 'telling it as it is' (see Chapter 6).

Nursing time and nursing space

In searching the evidence concerning the concepts of nursing time and nursing space, and not just time and space of itself, I came across both theoretical discussion papers and ethnographic studies in which they had been bound together. This section will focus on some of these as illustration of possibilities for nursing research. (Further examples of how time and space are seen in nursing culture will be seen in Chapters 5, 6, 7 and 10).

Brown & Brooks' (2002) study considered the 'temporal landscape of night nursing', which Brooks & MacDonald (2000) explored as a night-nursing subculture.

Their study was undertaken as a 'longitudinal ethnographic research' and in their conclusion they believe they had through this research arrived at a map – 'of the temporal landscape inhabited by night nurses as they go about their working lives' (p. 384). Their findings focused on 'three domains of temporal experience and perceptions, namely shift work, workload and temporal aspects of caring' (p. 386).

There are some valuable narratives by the nurses to illustrate each one of these. Shift work was found in time spans as described by Zerubavel, with the night shift being the longest in a 24-hour day. Here is a wonderful example of the 'temporal landscape', as experienced by someone who worked only night-duty shifts, and is one that I can certainly relate to as I worked as a Night Sister for a number of years:

> I come on at 8.30 and take report. There is a visual handover and there are usually two of us. We go round the beds and say hello to all the patients. The nurse from the day staff will tell me what has happened with that patient during the day. It doesn't take that long. About 5.30 in the morning you go round to make sure the patients are clean and tidy and they have slept okay. You do the handover to the day staff at 7.00 in the morning (Bernadette, 6 years on nights) (Brown & Brooks 2002, p. 387).

We can also see the way in which that night shift is ordered in terms of an activity, including this notion of the 'handover' of the patients' experience during the day and then the same in the morning. This activity I had discovered was part of a much larger system of communication that nurses relied on to carry out their work on a daily basis (Holland 1993). Philpin (2006) also focused on the concept of 'Handing Over', using anthropological insights to explore its meaning through ritual and symbolism. She cites the work of Zerubavel (1979a, p. 55) in relation to handovers and time – in that 'nursing duties and responsibilities are either assumed or suspended. Reports have a tremendous moral significance for nurses ....' (More detailed discussion of handovers as ritual and the work of Philpin will be discussed in Chapter 5.)

Seneviratne et al. (2009) undertook ethnographic fieldwork on a Canadian stroke unit, where they focused on 'nurses perceptions of the contexts of caring for acute stroke survivors'. They concluded that 'understanding how care providers conceive of and respond to space, time and *interprofessionalism has the potential to improve stroke care'* (p. 1872). In terms of space they arrived at some interesting themes: *'nursing in a submarine, nursing too close and nursing in a state of code burgundy'* (p. 1875). For the nurses in the unit the idea of being in a submarine related to their feeling of claustrophobia due to their perception that there was a lack of work and storage space. This was also related to the second theme of 'nursing too close' where the nurses had limited space to move about and also assure patient privacy amongst other things. The 'code burgundy' issue related to the name given to lack of beds and an extra bed in the hallway (a meaning I would read as the ward corridor) where again this provided an *'ethical challenge of hallway care'* to patients. Time in this study was seen as: 'lack of space, preserving time' and 'time with and without space'. Their finding in relation to the latter theme was that *'time and space were evolving and interconnected concepts'* (p. 1876) and that because of limited time and space, rehabilitation was hard to do on the unit itself. It also impacted on bedside rounds, given their multidisciplinary approach of various professions' input into the discussion of patients' care around the bedside.

An interesting study by Wakefield (2002) focused on the 'changing shape of the nurses' station' which in fact had been seen as a major barrier to effective working in the Seneviratne et al. (2009) study as well. The nursing station is a structure in the ward, and in fact has been present in one form or another since the Florence Nightingale development based on the concept invented in France, known as the Pavilion design which became known as the Nightingale ward (Forty 1980, pp. 78–79). In the early wards the Sister's office had a window overlooking the ward where all the patients could be observed or in Foucault's terms were 'under surveillance' (Foucault 2003). A similarity to this remains in place, as I personally experienced recently when I was admitted to a hospital ward and was placed in a four-bed ward immediately opposite the nurses' station which was also used as a focal point for all health care professionals coming and going on the ward (see p. 54). This time, however, I was under surveillance from the outside through the glass window next to my bed space.

Halford & Leonard (2003) talked about 'movement in space', that is how nurses they were observing in their research used their bodies within the ward space as well as the wider hospital space. One particular observation of theirs which I had experienced during my own observation or 'reverse gaze', that patients undertake to make the day time meaningful, is the way in which *'nurses move quickly, with purpose but in chore-driven ways – always busy, always doing something, buzzing around repetitive spatial patterns, communicating with each other in passing, snatched conversations'* (p. 204). They also found that different spaces had different meanings for nurses, and in which they acted differently, especially in relation to their own gendered identity. Nurses were also more restricted in their movement as they were ward based, whereas the doctors observed had more freedom to roam (p. 201).

Jones (2001) set out to explore the meaning of nursing time as he believed that, despite it being *'one of the most important influences on nursing behaviour'* (p. 150), it was not very visible in the literature. One major finding of his study was that he *'proposed that nurses exist and practice within nonlinear, complex and parallel worlds'*. But as we have already discussed, this is not in line with Hall's monochronic model of time which governs their normal monochronic workplaces.

Nursing time is also the focus to this work by Jones (2010) who has developed a framework for how this is seen and acted out. He states that because the practice of nursing takes place *'within a nursing work environment embedded in the sociocultural context of the health-care organisation'*, it creates in fact a *'dual role for the practising nurse, i.e. patient care provider and organisational employee'* (p. 185).

He explores initially how an understanding of time is informed by a number of disciplines, namely '*physics, psychology and sociology*' (p. 186). His framework is actually based around concepts from these three disciplines, to establish a single conceptual framework which is a 'work in progress'. In a later study (Jones 2015) he reports on the evaluation of a new instrument for '*measuring sociological nursing time*' and describes how this is experienced in nurses employed in a hospital. The focus of nursing work in relation to employment and also how it relates to others in the workplace will be discussed in more detail in Chapter 8. In brief, Jones (2010) defines these three nursing (work) times as follows:

> **Physical nursing time** is measured by the clock and assigned a number. It is exemplified by commonly used staffing metrics such as hours of care and nurse/patient ratios (p. 191).
>
> **Psychological nursing time** is conceived as that internal to providers and recipients of nursing care. It is subjective, perceptual and elastic. Psychological nursing time is influenced by the history, experience and expectations of the participants. It is what participants experience as nursing and how they experience it (p. 192).
>
> **The sociological form of nursing time** is therefore described as that which is experienced by providers and recipients of nursing care through shared temporal structures. It is a shared intersubjective experience of patterns of behaviour. Sociological nursing time is characterised by the sequential ordering of events within the daily routine of a practice setting (p. 192).

We can see in each of these definitions elements of what has already been explored earlier in this chapter and which will also resonate with your experiences, and most importantly it has to be remembered that according to Jones (2010, p. 191), '*Nursing time is also experienced within the social context of the healthcare system*', and all three elements of his proposed framework for exploring nursing time have to be considered against this background, and also most importantly how they also work together. There will always be commonalities in terms of the overall principles regarding nursing time across all health care systems but there will be an impact as to how these are then translated into the practice work of nurses. Two of the most important of these will be the political and cultural contexts in which nurses work.

Conclusion

This chapter has offered a short introduction to these major anthropological concepts of time and space (temporality and spatiality) but we can see from the literature discussed how important understanding their existence is in terms of nursing care and work. To understand their impact on nursing practice it is important not to forget the way in which nursing has itself developed over a period of time, from before Florence Nightingale in places such as Kaiserworth with daily routines governed by specific time slots, to the work of Florence Nightingale herself and her major interest in the design of hospital buildings and wards, especially in relation to public health and well-being. We will continue to explore aspects of these two major concepts of time and space in other chapters.

References

Antonacopoulou E P (2002) *Learning as Space: Implications for Organisational Learning*. Paper presented to the Third European Conference in Organisational Knowledge, Learning and Capabilities, Athens Laboratory of Business Administration, 5–6 April 2002.

Brooks I and Macdonald S (2000) 'Doing life': Gender relations in a night nursing sub-culture, *Gender, Work and Organisation*, 7(4), 221–229.

Brown R B & Brooks I (2002) The temporal landscape of night nursing, *Journal of Advanced Nursing*, 39 (4), 384–390.

Bullough B & Bullough V L (1964) *The Emergence of Modern Nursing*, Macmillan, New York.

Dorcy K S (1992) Built space and the socialization of nursing students, *Western Journal of Nursing Research*, 14(5), 632–644.

Forty A (1980) The modern hospital in England and France: The social and medical uses of architecture. In A D King (ed), *Buildings and Society: Essays on the Social Development of the Built Environment*, 61–93, Routledge, London.

Foucault M (2003) *The Birth of the Clinic*, Routledge Classics, Routledge, London.

Giger J N & Davidhizar R E (2008) *Transcultural Nursing, Assessment and Intervention*, 5th Edition, Mosby Elsevier, St Louis.

Gray P (2004) *Spatiality and the Lives of Student Nurses*, Unpublished PhD study, University of Stirling, Stirling.

Grint K (2005) *The Sociology of Work: Introduction*, Polity Press, Cambridge.

Halford S & Leonard P (2003) Space and place in the construction and performance of gendered nursing identities, *Journal of Advanced Nursing*, 42(2) 201–208.

Hall E T (1984) *The Dance of Life: The Other Dimensions of Time*, Anchor Books, New York.

Helman C (1992) Heart disease and the cultural construction of time. In R Frankenberg (ed), *Time, Health and Medicine*. Sage, London.

Henderson V (1960) *Basic Principles of Nursing Care*, International Council of Nurses, Geneva.

Henderson V (1991) *The Nature of Nursing: Reflections after 25 Years*, National League for Nursing, New York.

Hockey J (1990) *Experiences of Death: An Anthropological Account*, Edinburgh University Press, Edinburgh.

Holland C K (1993) An ethnographic study of nursing culture as an exploration for determining the existence of a system of ritual, *Journal of Advanced Nursing*, 18, 1461–1470.

Holland K (1999) A journey to becoming: The student nurse in transition, *Journal of Advanced Nursing*, 29(1), 1461–1470.

Jones A (2001) Time to think: Temporal considerations in nursing practice and research, *Journal of Advanced Nursing*, 32(2), 150–158.

Jones T L (2010) A holistic framework for nursing time: Implications for theory, practice and research, *Nursing Forum*, 45(3), 185–196.

Jones T L (2015) Dimensions of nurse work time: Progress in instrumentation, *Nursing & Health Sciences*, 17, 323–330.

Jowsey T, Yen L & Mathews P (2012) Time spent on health related activities associated with chronic illness: A scoping literature review, *BMC Public Health*, 12(1044)

Lawler J (1991) *Behind the screens: Nursing, Somology and the Problem of the Body*, Churchill Livingstone, Edinburgh.

Littlewood J (1991) Care and ambiguity: Towards a concept of nursing. In P Holden & J Littlewood (1991) *Anthropology and Nursing*, Chapter 10, 170–189, Routledge, London.

Manthey M (1980) *The Practice of Primary Nursing*, Blackwell Scientific Publications, Boston. PhilpinS M (2006) 'Handing over': Transmission of information between nurses in an intensive therapy unit, *Nursing in Critical Care*, 11(2), 86–93.

Roth J A (1963) *Timetables: Structuring the Passage of Time in Hospital Treatment and other Careers*, The Bobbs-Merrill Company, Indianapolis.

Royal College of Nursing (2014) *Defining Nursing*, RCN, London.

Savage J (1995) *Nursing Intimacy: An Ethnographic Approach to Nurse-Patient Interaction*, Scutari Press, London.

Seneviratne C C, Mather M & Then K L (2009) Understanding nursing on an acute stroke unit: Perceptions of space, time and interprofessional practice, *Journal of Advanced Nursing*, 65(9), 1872–1881.

Shebini N, Aggarwal R & Gandhi A (2008) Improved patient awareness of named nursing through audit, *Nursing Times*, 104(21), 30–31.

Smith C W (1972) *Florence Nightingale*, Book Club Associates, London.

Strauss A, Schatzman L, Ehrlich D, Bucher R & Sabshin M (1963) The hospital and its negotiated order. In E Freidson (ed), *The Hospital in Modern Society*, 147–169, Free Press of Glencoe, New York.

Twigg J (1999) The spatial ordering of care: Public and private in bathing support at home, *Sociology of Health and Illness*, 21(4), 381–400.

Van Maanen J (1988) *Tales of the Field: On Writing Ethnography*, 2nd Edition, University of Chicago Press, Chicago.

Wakefield A (2002) The changing 'shape' of the nursing station, *Contemporary Nurse*, 13(2–3), 148–157.

Wolf Z R (1988) *Nurses' Work: The Sacred and the Profane*, University of Pennsylvania, Pennsylvania.

Zerubavel E (1979a) *Patterns of Time in Hospital Life: A Sociological Perspective*, University of Chicago Press, Chicago.

Zerubavel E (1979b) The temporal organisation of continuity: The case of medical and nursing coverage, *Human Organisation*, 38(1), 78–83.

Zerubavel E (1981) *Hidden Rhythms: Schedules and Calendars in Social Life*, University of Chicago Press, Chicago. 1st California Press Paperback Edition published in 1985.

Further reading

1   Andrews G J (2003) Locating a geography of nursing: Space, place and the progress of geographical thought, *Nursing Philosophy*, 4, 231–248.

2   Andrews G J & Shaw D (2008) Clinical geography: Nursing practice and the (re) making of institutional space, *Journal of Nursing Management*, 16, 463–473.

3   Caldas C P (2012) A concept analysis about temporality and its applicability in nursing care, *Nursing Forum*, 47(4), 245–252.

4   Chapple H S (2010) *No Place for Dying: Hospitals and the Ideology of Rescue*, Left Coast Press.

5   Coleman S & Collins P (2006) *Locating the Field – Space, Place and Context in Anthropology*, Berg, Oxford.

6   Dalton L M (2004) Time as a source of conflict: Student nurse experiences of clinical practice in a rural setting, *The International Electronic Journal of Rural and Remote Health Research, Education, Practice and Policy*, 256, 1–10.

7   Fox N J Power, control and resistance in the timing of health and care, *Social Science and medicine*, 48(10), 1307–1319.

8   Frankenberg R (ed) (1992) *Time, Health and Medicine*, Sage Publications, London.

9   Freidson E (1963) *The Hospital in Modern Society*, The Free Press of Glencoe, London.

10 Gesler W M & Kearns R A (2002) *Culture, Place and Health*, Routledge, London.

11 Giger J N (2016) *Transcultural Nursing, Assessment and Intervention*, 7th Edition, Elsevier, St Louis.

12 Gilmour J A (2005) Hybrid space: Constituting the hospital as a home space for patients, *Nursing Inquiry*, 13(1), 16–22.

13 Glaser B G & Strauss A L (1968) *Time for Dying*, Aldine Transaction, Chicago.

14 Goddard H (1953) *The Work of Nurses in Hospital wards. Report of a Job-Analysis*, Nuffield Provincial Hospitals Trust, London.

15 Golander H (1995) Rituals of temporality: The social construction of time in a nursing ward, *Journal of Aging Studies*, 9(2), 119–135.

16 Hall E T (1990) *The Hidden Dimension*, Anchor Books, New York.

17 Hockey J, KomaromyC & WoodthorpeK (2010) *The Matter of Death: Space, Place and Materiality*, Palgrave Macmillan, Basingstoke.

18   Richardson R (2010) Florence Nightingale and hospital design (http://www.kingscollections.org/exhibitions/specialcollections/nightingale-and-hospital-design/florence-nightingale-and-hospital-design, accessed 6 May 2019).

19   Savage J (1997) Gestures of resistance: The nurse's body in contested space, *Nursing Inquiry*, 4, 237–245.

20   Savishinsky J S (1991) *The Ends of Time: Life and Work in a Nursing Home*, Bergen & Garvey, New York.

21   Zerubavel E (1976) Timetables and scheduling: On the social organization of time, *Sociological Inquiry*, 46(2), 87–94.

22   Zerubavel E (1987) The Language of time: Towards a semiotics of temporality, *The Sociological Quarterly*, 28(3), 343–356.

5

RITUALS, RITES AND NURSING PRACTICE

Karen Holland

Introduction

In determining that nursing is a culture, it is logical to consider that, as in other cultures, there will be some kind of ritual practice in evidence. My own interest, as shown in Chapter 2, began with this question of whether there could be considered to be a ritual system in nursing culture. Through exploration of a ward setting using an ethnographic research design, I concluded that given my findings at that time, there were indeed rituals found in that field of study. This chapter uses that as its premise, and explores first the definition of ritual as used in anthropology followed by related aspects of a ritual that can be seen in transition and initiation contexts as related to nursing specifically. These are often known as rites of passage or in sociological literature as status passage; both will be considered in relation to student nurses, in particular in Chapter 6. This was the focus of later research on the initiation of student nurses (Holland 1999).

Rituals found by researchers in the context of nursing practice will also be explored, in particular those that have an impact on the delivery of care by nurses in different clinical contexts. These include rituals related to death and dying, observations, nursing care such as bathing patients and the ward or nursing handover. As it is not possible to explore the wider anthropological studies that involve ritual practice I have included some of these in the Further Reading section. Readers can then expand their knowledge base and consider some of the issues discussed in relation to this chapter from a wider range of literature.

Ritual and initiation

La Fontaine (1985, p. 11) describes ritual as 'social action' whereby its performance involves shared meaning and co-operative enactment by individuals, '*directed by a leader or leaders*'. There are rules of inclusion and exclusion and despite some change to the actual ritual procedure there is a '*sense that ritual has a fixed structure*' (p. 11). The rules of exclusion are '*of as much significance as those which permit or require others to take part*' (p. 11). La Fontaine stresses that: '*conventional behaviour, however regularly repeated, is not ritual*'.

Schultz & Lavenda's (2013, p. 57) definition strengthens the view expressed by La Fontaine and identifies ritual as consisting of four elements to its enactment:

> is composed of a sequence of symbolic activities, set off from the social routines of everyday life, recognisable by members of the society as a ritual and closely connected to a specific set of ideas often encoded in myth. What gives rituals their power is that participants assert that the authorisation for the ritual comes from outside themselves – from the state, society, God, the ancestors, or 'tradition'.

We can consider then that ritual is therefore action – and how it is performed is as meaningful as its purpose.

The link between ritual and initiation is embodied in the ritual performance known as 'rites of passage', which are a set of rituals which mark the moving and transforming of individuals from one status position to another (La Fontaine 1985; Van Gennep 1960). Van Gennep identified three stages within such rituals – separation, transition and incorporation. If we adopt the premise that ritual is action which has a predetermined text, then the performance within each stage of the rites of passage should be clearly visible.

Victor Turner (1969) extended Van Gennep's work and focused on the change in social status which occurs with a ritual performance. Both Turner and Van Gennep's work focuses on an anthropological meaning to ritual with its prescriptive nature, as opposed to Glaser & Strauss (1971) who, as sociologists, appeared to presume that although there were specific set properties to 'rites of passage' they were not as prescriptive as previously thought. They were in fact more flexible in relation to the social changes taking place around them. Their work, as with other sociologists, focused especially on *status passages that occur within occupations and within organizations* (p.2).

It could be argued therefore that Glaser & Strauss (1971) in fact focus mainly on the nature of the status passage itself, whilst Turner (1969) focused on the processes involved in the transition rituals, for example, what happens to the actual participants, that is the enactment of the ritual performance. A status is, for Glaser and Strauss, not a permanent position for an individual, and at some stage in time this will change, either willingly as part of a planned action or unwillingly by being 'dispossessed' of that status (1971, p. 3).

Whether it is Van Gennep's *The Rites of Passage* or Glaser and Strauss's *Status Passage*, there are key elements that have an impact on what takes place; these are the temporal, spatial and cultural conditions in which they exist. From these three, temporality appears to take the major share of influence in relation to the nature and occupation of a passage from one status to another (p. 33). This will be further explored in Chapter 6.

The purpose of ritual in society in functionalist terms could be to maintain social cohesion and social order in society, which is reflected in Turner's view of ritual as a social phenomenon, that is: *'a periodic restatement of the terms in which men of a particular culture must interact if there is to be any kind of coherent social life'*.

Helman (2007) states that Turner sees the two inherent functions of rituals he describes as expressive and creative. The expressive function is one that symbolically communicates certain lay values and culture articulates and experiences these in a dramatic form. The creative function, however, *'actually creates or re-creates the categories through which men perceive reality, the axioms underlying the structure of society and the laws of the natural and moral orders'* (Helman 2007, p. 225).

On reading both Van Gennep and Turner's work as well as Bell (1992; 1997) it is clear that there is one major aspect of rituals that we need to consider, and we will look at this later in relation to ritual in nursing, and that is the use of symbols. A symbol in basic terms is *'something which is used to represent an idea or object'* (Pountney & Maric 2015, p17) and when we see these symbols placed together or used together they can have a shared meaning for a community.

For example, nurses seeing a photo of a nurse (Florence Nightingale) in her traditional uniform, holding a lamp set against the background of images of soldiers, will consider the symbolism of all three 'objects' – the person in the uniform, the lamp and the injured soldiers – to reflect not only the work of Nightingale herself but that of nursing and caring for the wounded as well as sacrifice on the part of nurses who volunteered to work in the dangerous conditions in the Crimean war.

Ritual and initiation are linked, in that rituals are enacted in order to enable the participants to undertake a clearly marked transition in society that is recognised by other social groups. However, the initiation from one social group to another does not include the transmission of knowledge and powers that are exclusive to the initiated.

In relation to the student nurse, for example, this knowledge and power will only be as allowed by the professional body that is the Nursing and Midwifery Council or its equivalent in another country. An excellent example of what this initiation does not include in the new NMC 2018 Standards of Proficiency is the ability of the student nurse, on transition to the new role of qualified nurse, *to prescribe certain medication*, as had been originally intended (Nursing and Midwifery Council 2018). This power to prescribe will rest with the nurse when the transition to registered nurse has been made and only then after another short programme will the newly qualified nurse be allowed to prescribe from a very limited formulary.

There is also according to Loudan a public and a private element to ritual (Loudan 1966) – the public being more evidence of the symbolism associated with ritual enactment – and where there is visible evidence of the participants undergoing initiation or transitional state, for example different uniforms. The private action of ritual is that closely related to the knowledge that is acquired through the initiation process, and it is found within those rituals associated with one person or social groups, where, for example, their status within society is marked, such as in age-related groups. For the student nurse this could be related to their actual year groups or when they began their transition from pre-student nurse given a group number, or set number as identified by MacGuire (1968), which differentiated them from the group in front of them or those coming after them. In addition, they will be given a different stripe on their uniform in some organisations to represent their year group – or similar stage in those groups – which we can take to be akin to age groups in tribal societies (see Chapter 6).

Many rituals can also be found associated with different religions and their performance related to what one calls the sacred as opposed to the secular in the world (Pountney & Maric 2015, p. 163). We can see this in the way that some religions, such as Muslim, have to undertake certain activities which act as a kind of purification of the body. These can involve *'washing hands, face, arms and feet with water'* before prayers. Of course, in a hospital these same activities may not be possible so patients are enabled to adapt these and ensure that they complete as many as possible, especially if they are restricted to their bed area (Holland 2017).

The main rituals we are looking at in this chapter are non-religious rituals as they relate to nursing.

However, given its strong link with being considered a religious 'calling' and vocation there remains a religious aspect to nursing, especially some nursing celebrations or rites celebrating the life of Florence Nightingale. The annual service that takes place in Westminster Abbey, London, for example, where a chosen small group of nurses accompany one Nursing Sister who carries the symbolic lamp of Florence Nightingale, is one such 'ritual', imbued with ritual action and religious meaning. The nurses are all dressed in various uniforms and include the wearing of the nurses' hats representing the different status of nurse. (See this example from 2018: https://www.westminster-abbey.org/abbey-news/florence-nightingale-remembered and the order of service which explains the conduct of the service: https://www.westminster-abbey.org/media/8592/florence-nightingale-2018-service.pdf as well as further information from the Florence Nightingale Foundation: https://florence-nightingale-foundation.org.uk/about/westminster-abbey-commemoration-service/.)

The wearing of hats is no longer seen in UK hospitals nor many other countries, due to many reasons including infection control and a desire to see nurses relinquish past practices. However, hats are worn for this 'religious' ceremony which takes place annually in one of the most revered of places associated with religion, and with the same order to the service, which includes the carrying of the lamp as a symbol associated with Florence Nightingale.

Bates (2010) has published a wonderful article on *The Nurse's Cap and its Rituals*, including the traditional 'capping ceremony' for Canadian student nurses who had survived their six-month probation. Being given a cap was a mark of transition from their probationary period and a symbol of their ongoing journey to becoming a nurse. It is worth reading a brief explanation by Bates of this ceremony as it relates to this chapter and the previous example of what is still celebrated:

> For the student nurse, the capping ceremony provided a deep sense of validation and belonging. In a conflation of quasi-religious and nursing folklore, probationary students accepted into the nursing programme would stand or kneel to receive their caps, light candles or lamps as symbols of nursing, and recite the Florence Nightingale pledge, this transcendent ceremony with its special place, dress, gesture and rhetoric had all the characteristics of ritual in the anthropological sense, and in particular, of a rite of passage. It was a call to the higher purpose of caring as well as legitimation of the hierarchical system of nursing education (p. 33).

Bates (2012) has also written a book on *A Cultural History of the Nurse's Uniform* where the capping ceremony is included along with aspects of the history of nursing and the day-to-day lives of student and qualified nurses. In particular we can see the transition from the traditional uniform of dress, apron and cap to the more casual form of dress described as 'scrubs', which I always recall as being worn by nurses and doctors in the operating theatre or intensive care units. We can see in the UK health service today, the development of this less 'traditional nursing look' and the option for student nurses and staff nurses to wear tops and trousers for working in practice areas, and by doing so, from my own personal experience, this often contributes to the confusion for patients of who is a student nurse or a qualified nurse amongst all the health care workers in a hospital. Differentiation amongst staff is now through the use of colour – either as different bands on a white background or different-coloured tops, or in the case of qualified nurses different-coloured dresses for different statuses of nursing staff (see Chapter 6).

Routine and ritual

One issue that does need clarifying before we consider rituals in nursing specifically is the difference between routine and ritual. Pountney & Maric (2015) offer a succinct definition of these two:

> Routines are one-dimensional in meaning, whereas rituals have multi-level meanings. For example, brushing your teeth, washing your hands, eating and going to sleep at night are routines. However the same actions can become ritual if certain symbolic actions are involved (p. 164).

This difference is a very important one to consider in relation to nursing practice, as some authors (Walsh & Ford 1989) have given different nursing activities a ritual title but in fact they do not contain clear symbolic attributes or meaning nor do they meet the initial definition of a ritual as defined by La Fontaine and other anthropologists. It is worth mentioning their book at this point, because in their view the traditions and history of nursing aligned with the domination of the hospitals and medical establishments (p. ix) were causing nurses to fail patients and therefore themselves. They considered that: '*The cause of this failure we suggest, is rooted in the traditional rituals and myths that still abound in the wards and departments of today*' (p. ix).

The book then proceeded to explain away that, because of the fact that nurses continued to practice as they had always been doing and not based on any clear evidence base, all these practices were rituals. One example focused on pre-operative preparation of the patient, whereby they stated that: '*In view of the overwhelming amount of evidence there is no place for the traditional skin shave as part of pre-op preparation. It is a ritual based on a myth*' (p. 8).

There are many similar deliberations throughout the whole book but no clear definition is offered as to what they mean and define as ritual and ritualistic practice. A statement about nursing report as a ritual at the start of the day on a ward is not without some validity if considered in a broader context (Holland 1993); however, Walsh & Ford (1989) then denigrate this possibility with their view that: '*We have an inefficient system which is a hangover from the past; in other words, a ritual*' (p. 119).

Even student nurses at the time were considered guilty of ritualistic practice: '*Another ritual involves the little nursing notebooks in which students usually desperately scribble notes in the hope of being able to retain some shreds of information relevant to their patients*' (p. 119).

We need to be reminded that this work was published at a time when the pursuit of new nursing practices such a the nursing process, primary nursing, evidence-based practice and avoidance of such nursing practices as task-focused patient care were being advocated. Nevertheless many of their statements throughout, which have no clear foundation by which we can compare using a clear definition of their initial meaning of ritual and ritualistic behaviour or practice, remain concerning, not just from a nursing practice point of view but because they encourage an ongoing belief that a great deal of nursing practice becomes ritualistic and that rituals in nursing are therefore bad for nursing.

Philpin (2002) also notes this view of Walsh & Ford (1989; 1994) on ritual action, '*as carrying out a task without thinking it through in a problem-solving way. The nurse does something because this is the way it has always been done*' (p. 9), which she argues '*ignores the meaning and purpose of many nursing actions*' (p. 144). Philpin (2004) in her PhD research study considered ritual and symbolism in an intensive therapy unit and her 2002 paper focused on much of the literature on ritual, offering a balanced critique on much of what I have already referenced in this chapter, including my own initial, possibly naïve, exploration into considering whether ritual in nursing culture existed. Philpin's (2006) main finding in her fieldwork was that:

> whilst nursing work in this ITU was undoubtedly grounded in evidence-based practice, elements of symbolism and ritual were also an integral part of the nurses' work and their work environment. That is to argue that these two, seemingly contradictory aspects of nursing work, coexisted in this unit (p. ii).

You may consider this next statement of Walsh & Ford (1989) against what you know of nursing practice today and also return to it when you have read the rest of the book:

> Qualified staff who do not keep up to date with research findings have little other than intuition, outdated teaching, ritual and mythology to guide their practice. While there may be a place for intuition in the art of nursing, there is no place in the science of nursing for ritual and mythology! (p. x).

We have no space here to debate this view of intuition and whether nursing is an art or a science, but the distinct lack of theoretical underpinning evidence and knowledge related to both ritual and mythology in the context of nursing as a developing profession and discipline was a concern at the time of first reading the book. The omission, for example, even briefly, of the major work by two American researchers who had undertaken studies directly related to nursing and ritualistic practices already was unexplained. As we will see the work by Virginia Walker in 1967 and later Zane Robinson Wolf (1986a; 1988a; 1988b) was highly relevant to any discussion of nursing rituals, whether to dispute or defend their value in relation to the development of an evidence-based-practice nursing profession.

Despite referencing the work of Christine Chapman (1983) on 'Ritual and rational action in hospitals' and the work of Isabel Menzies (1960) on how nurses manage stressful situations by using defensive actions there is no exploration of their relationship to their own examination of nursing rituals. Philpin (2002) also makes reference to this omission and Silberger (1998) cautions that Walsh & Ford (1989) misused the terms 'mythology' and 'myths' when describing '*procedures and patient care interactions*'.

Chapman (1983) made it very clear how she saw rituals differently to Menzies as she undertook her participant observation in a number of London hospitals and sought to compare Menzies' (1960) 'Ritual Task Performance: Psychodynamic Model' with her own 'Ritual and Rational Action: Sociological model'. Chapman's observations focused on a range of rituals such as greeting rituals, concealment rituals and hospital-specific lifecycle rituals. Examples of these such as those associated with managing the death of a patient on a ward and other hospital units are of particular importance because many of these remain with us today.

Glaser & Strauss (1965; 1968) who Chapman cites in relation to dying in hospital see the situation as having a certain trajectory where there are specific rituals associated with each stage. She observed, in relation to nursing practice, the screening of the dead patient from sight of others on the ward, followed then by a procedure known by nurses as 'last offices', where the dead patient was washed, clothed in a white gown and then encased in a white sheet (see Chapter 7). Following this personal care every other patient on the ward was then screened from seeing the dead patient being removed from the ward on a mortuary trolley which was also covered by a sheet. Following this removal of the dead person from the ward, all screens were pushed back, the bed cleaned and eventually remade. No one said anything to the remaining patients about what had been happening but from my own personal experiences of nurse training in the late 1960s onwards patients spoke quietly amongst themselves and drew the right conclusions. Nurses often had to comfort patients following such situations in particular if they had developed a strong patient–patient relationship with the deceased person. Certainly in the 1960s and 1970s this would happen, as patients stayed in hospital for longer periods of time than today. The fear that they would also succumb to a similar fate was at these times paramount in their minds.

This separation of the dead from the living remains a nursing practice, as seen in Templeman's (2015) ethnography in the ICU (see Chapter 9) where the curtains were drawn around the patient who was either in a transition state after a decision to withdraw treatment or had already died, and which offered space for the patient's relatives to grieve.

Rituals and symbols

Rituals are always associated with symbolic action and symbols (Douglas 1996) which we will find in certain aspects of nursing practice, both past and present. These include those associated with death and dying in various nursing contexts as seen by Chapman (1983), the symbolism associated with becoming a qualified nurse with regards to uniforms, caps and celebration of passing examinations, and the change from being a student to becoming a qualified nurse and those actions that are involved in this rite of passage or transition from one stage and status to another (see Chapter 6).

Helman (2007) pointed out that:

> Although Turner's concept of ritual symbols concentrated mostly on physical objects, there are many other components of ritual that can also be regarded as having strong symbolic value. When included in a ritual they can signal important information to both participants and observers (p. 225).

It is important that these other possible components within a ritual are mentioned here in the context of ritual as both a performance and as a transition, because we will see that many are relevant in our personal lives as well as professional lives with many being very important to the health and illness, as well as religious, belief systems of patients we meet in the context of nursing work. It is also important to be aware that they have different meanings in different cultures (Holland 2017).

Helman notes some of these as:

> **clothing** (such as a nurse's uniform or doctor's white coat); **colours** (black for mourning and death in one culture and white in another); **body decorations** (body art such as an Indian bride's hands and feet are covered in henna designs); **smell** (such as incense in

a church or temple); **tastes** (certain drinks that are used within a ritual – the tea ceremony); **foods** (a wedding cake); **sounds** (chanting or bells); **words** (specific words said during a prayer or at a nurse's graduation ceremony in some countries); **silences** (essential periods of silence in a religious service such as a burial); **rhythms** (music that has meaning during a wedding service); **movements** (a tribal dance) and **gestures** (**crossing oneself on entering a church**) (Helman 2007, p. 225 – Helman's words are in bold).

All rituals have a temporal and spatial context set in the specific cultural context in which they exist. We can first consider these as related to a transition or passage.

Rites of passage

The work of Arnold Van Gennep, an early French anthropologist, has become the major source of information about ritual as it applies to the moving from one life status to another in a series of stages. These have symbolic meaning and many have associated celebrations or ceremonies. One that comes to mind here are those rites associated with marriage, from a single status in life to that of being engaged then married, with all the respective symbolism and rituals associated with these stages in life as seen in countries like the UK. Similar rituals are also associated with this single-to-marriage state in smaller-scale societies such as tribal cultures of the world.

As already seen in previous sections the rites of passage as defied by Van Gennep have three key stages, with a major focus on the actual stage of transition itself called liminality.

These stages are: **A separation stage** from a previous situation or way of life; **the transition stage** where the initiate (given that this whole ritual is called an initiation – as per La Fontaine – those who participate are known as initiates) is not at one stage or another, and called the liminal or marginal stage. This stage for the student nurse is where they learn to become a qualified nurse through various steps or 'tests' to go through; the third stage then becomes that of **incorporation**, where the initiate then enters society in a new position or status, with of course new role expectations. This is usually marked in some way by another rite, which Holland (1999) found was the awarding of the registration by the Nursing and Midwifery Council to acknowledge that the student nurse was now a registered nurse and entitled to use the title of nurse.

However, as we will see in Chapter 6, Holland (1999, p. 235) discovered in her study that there was a period towards the end of their transition to this registration where the student nurses found themselves 'in social limbo' at two different times – once before the students left college after their course of study ended, and again before they received their registration acknowledgement by the then UKCC.

Their official transition had to wait, but she found that their social transition and completion and ending of their student nurse status was marked by graduation social event but their official graduation from the university and their academic and practice awards had to wait until much later. Other researchers such as Kath Melia (1987) had acknowledged that students in her study also found this transition experience to be a stressful time, and that uncertainty and concerns about being able to cope with their new nursing status as a qualified nurse was clearly an issue. Further literature and discussion about rites of passage and initiation will be explored in Chapter 6.

Nursing rituals

In order to establish how ritual is seen in the nursing literature I have chosen to focus on those associated with specific themes from my own research and those of others, to ensure that the major works are highlighted. We can look at the broad literature initially in terms of how authors have perceived rituals in relation to nursing practice beyond what we have already discussed. Although there is a developed body of research literature (Walker 1967; Wolf 1986a; Wolf 1988b; Wolf 1997; Holland 1993; Philpin 2004; Philpin 2006; Lee 2001; Goopy 2005; Jiyane et al. 2012; O'Gorman 1998) related to nursing rituals it is not significant to have created a major interest in exploring nursing practice for evidence of its presence. There are other papers that focus on exploring the literature on rituals as they relate to nursing and offering their views and opinions on what evidence there is (DeLuca 1995; Biley & Wright 1997; Suominen et al. 1997; Silberger 1998; Strange 2001; Catanzaro 2002; Teres 1993; Philpin 2002; McAllister 2008; Wolf 2014).

I would like to begin this final discussion section with the work of Virginia Walker (1967) who had noticed a number of issues taking place in clinical practice around various nursing activities such as recording and charting observations and reporting on patients at change of shift time. The rationale for some of these was not clear. She notes that because of some of the practices involving both student nurses and qualified nurses, there could be a problem '*if busy nursing personnel found it necessary to perform these routines with little or no recognised value to the patient*' (p. 5); there needed to be more clarity as to why nurses carried them out. She was also very clear that how ritual was defined in these situations needed clarity and most important from my point of view was her statement that: '*Branding an activity as ritualistic does not make it, in and of itself, undesirable. Many so called rituals of daily life are a positive means of accomplishment, and if not materially productive, do contribute to the wellbeing of someone*' (p. 6).

To me reading this nearly 25 years later was very illuminating, and in particular that Walker was funded to study '*Ritualism in nursing and its effects on patient care*'.

Defining what was meant by ritualism became the first task. The need to have a definition that actually focused on the ritualistic behaviour of nurses in relation to practice meant that they excluded the use of 'ritualistic' related to codes or systems of rites and ceremonies – and expressive behaviour, to focus on a definition by Robert Merton (1956), whereby '*he refers to ritualism as patterns of response in which culturally defined aspirations are abandoned while one continues to abide almost compulsively by institutional norms*' (p. 7). However, Walker stressed that this did not explain everything that they had seen undertaken by nurses – such as continuing to take regular patient temperatures when not needed anymore. Eventually another definition was agreed for the study: '*ritualism refers to behaviour which has a special significance to the actor rather than orientation toward achieving organisational goals.*' She implied that this definition linked the actions to something that could reduce anxiety in a person or some other psychological need.

Their definition in fact very much related to that espoused by Isobel Menzies (1960) in her work on social defence systems and how student nurses in particular were encouraged to stick to prescribed behaviour when performing tasks in order that they learn to keep doing them correctly as 'a prescribed ritual'. Of course neither of these definitions meet that related specifically to an anthropological meaning but are essential reading in understanding how this early work led to the misunderstanding about task-centred care as being ritualistic practice which had no function other than it had 'always been done that way'. Walker studied a number of practices that had been defined as ritualistic by research participants: '*writing of nurses notes, the taking of temperatures, pulse and respiration, the functioning of the shift report, and the use of the special report*' (page 8). Without individualising all the findings here, suffice to say that her overall view is that what she found in her research '*did not provide a clear-cut picture of nurses dedicated to ritualistic practice*' but that there was strong argument for the fact that '*much behaviour with the nursing department is organisationally ineffective*' (p. 169). This of course had organisational outcomes required to enhance nursing practices and concluded that this was of more concern 'than if the data indicated more prevalent ritualistic practices' (p. 169). She concluded with an important statement which we will see in other research in relation to value of rituals, whereby: '*Rituals, at least, have a meaning for the performer*'.

Focusing on similar areas of care to Walker (1967), Zane Robinson Wolf carried out an ethnographic study for her doctorate (Wolf 1986b) which focused on 'Nursing rituals in an adult acute care hospital' (see: https://repository.upenn.edu/dissertations/AAI8614888/). She later published her work as a book with a wonderful title: *Nurses' Work: The Sacred and The Profane* (Wolf 1988b). The definition of ritual she used in her study was that of De Craemer et al. (1976) which was: '*ritual is patterned symbolic action that refers to the goals and values of a social group*' (p. iv). She identified the main three therapeutic nursing rituals which were *post-mortem care, administration of medication* and *the bath* (in relation to aseptic practices and hygiene needs) and one occupational nursing ritual, which was the *Shift report*. The issue of admission and discharge of a patient from hospital she also considered as having patient ritual elements but her data did not find specific nursing beliefs and values specific to these procedures that could be called 'rituals' (Wolf 1988b). She also noted that '*nurses passed on subcultural knowledge by demonstration and by an oral tradition of information exchange*' (p. v).

Her PhD study reads as a written ethnography with narrated text which brings to life her observations and field notes. Her 'conceptual orientation' as she defines her literature review is steeped in the discussion of ritual from anthropology, sociology and nursing (p. 6), in particular Turner (1969) and his work related to '*the rituals of affliction performed by Ndembu healers*', Mary Douglas (1966) and her work in relation to symbolism of purity and those related to sacred and profane and pollution (Douglas 1975). The work of Van Gennep (1960) also influenced her thinking in relation to initiation rituals discussed in Chapter 6. Philpin (2007) also considered this issue of pollution in relation to what happens to various boundaries in the ITU environment, in particular in relation to the situation encountered by the nurses caring for patients in this environment. I will explore this concept further in Chapter 8.

As we have already seen, the work of Walker (1967) offered much food for thought in Wolf's work, and noted that the '*change of shift report seemed to serve professional nurses and the practical nurses as a means of maintaining group cohesion*' (p. 16). My own study (Holland 1993) had also experienced that the 'handover report' was of some significance, and that '"*reporting time" appeared to be a cultural rule, an unwritten law that all nurses should attend and it would appear to be a way of ensuring that social order is maintained within the group by enforcing cohesion and interaction*' (p. 1467). Wolf was very clear, however, that any preconceived ideas about what ritual was and whether it offered a positive or negative function should be avoided prior to studying it and that in her study what the concept of nursing ritual was became clear from her '*analysis of ethnographic data*' (p. 17).

My own exploration was to determine whether ritual existed in a nursing culture and, like Wolf (1986a), not whether it had a negative or positive function, just that it existed.

The Bath ritual, as well as being related to 'being clean', was also discussed by Wolf (1997) as a form of purification of the patient and removal of dirt in a clean environment, but most importantly she concluded that it met the definition by De Craemer et al. (1976) as therapeutic, and that this bathing of patients especially on admittance to hospital '*was performed to have a beneficial effect*'. The 'ritual of the bath' is explored further in Chapter 8. A shortened paper from her main study on nursing rituals was also published by Wolf (1988a) (see her paper which can be accessed in full from: cjnr.archive.mcgill.ca/article/download/ 1009/1009).

In terms of authors who have written about rituals without having undertaken actual research in the field, those noted at the beginning of this chapter offer various opinions from gathered evidence. I will be exploring more of these in later chapters such as Chapter 6: Transition and initiation; Chapter 8: Dirt, pollution and the body; Chapter 7: Nursing work within nursing culture.

However, as I end this chapter I would like to offer this view by Silberger (1998) concerning nursing, nursing culture and rituals as a way of pulling together what many of the authors we have considered here have alluded to, but also how it fits with many of the issues discussed in Chapters 1 and 2. It is not the whole of what Silberger explored in her article but offers a way of linking ritual as part of the wider culture of nursing but she also makes it clear that how nurses carry out their nursing and patient care practice mustn't be confused with the possible relevance that some nursing actions as rituals are an important and inherent part of the culture of nursing:

> Nursing is a cultural group that is defined by its group norms, values, attitudes, beliefs, rituals and ritualistic behaviour. Ritual defines part of the culture of nursing, but not nursing practice. Rituals in nursing culture strengthen the profession; perjoratively labelling nursing practice as 'ritualistic' undermines and weakens the profession. Ritual should not be confused with practice patterns (p. 12).

Conclusion

This chapter began with an attempt to bring together different meanings of ritual as seen in the wider anthropological literature and to consider how this has then been viewed in nursing as both practice and as a culture. A ritual, although a named action that may not be recognised as such by nurses in the course of their work, can exist alongside those activities that are simply carried out by nurses as part of their daily work and that are part of the different patterns of care that they give to patients in a variety of clinical settings. Rituals exist as part of the temporal, spatial and cultural contexts in which nursing takes place and are therefore an essential part of the tapestry that is woven over time to enable us to hold on to what is deemed important to retain as part of nursing's cultural heritage.

References

Bates C (2010) The Nurse's Cap and its Rituals, *The Journal of the Costume Society of America*, 36(1), 21–40.
Bates C (2012) *A Cultural History of the Nurse's Uniform*, Canadian Museum of Civilisations, Gatineau.
Bell C (1992) *Ritual Theory, Ritual Practice*, Oxford University Press, Oxford.
Bell C (1997) *Ritual Perspectives and Dimensions*, Oxford University Press, Oxford.

Biley F C & Wright S G (1997) Towards a defence of nursing routine and ritual, *Journal of Clinical Nursing*, 6, 115–119.

Catanzaro A M (2002) Beyond the misapprehension of nursing rituals, *Nursing Forum*, 37(2), 17–27.

Chapman G E (1983) Ritual and rational action in hospitals, *Journal of Advanced Nursing*, 8, 13–20.

DeLuca E K (1995) Reconsidering rituals: A vehicle for educational change, *The Journal of Continuing Education in Nursing*, 26(3), 139–144.

De Craemer W, Vansina J & Fox R (1976) Religious movements in Central Africa. *Comparative Studies in Society and History*, 18, 458–475.

Douglas M (1966) *Purity and Danger: An Analysis of Concept of Pollution and Taboo*, Routledge, London. Routledge Classic Edition published in 2002.

Douglas M (1975) Pollution. In M Douglas (ed), *Implicit Meanings: Essays in Anthropology*, 47–59, Routledge, London.

Douglas M (1996) *Natural Symbols: Exploration in Cosmology*, 2nd Edition, Routledge, London.

Glaser B G & StraussA L (1965) *Awareness of Dying*, Aldine, Chicago.

Glaser B G & StraussA L (1968) *Time for Dying*, Aldine Transaction, Chicago.

Glaser B G & StraussA L (1971) *Status Passage*, Aldine Transaction, New Brunswick.

Goopy S E (2005) Taking account of local culture: Limits to the development of a professional ethos, *Nursing Inquiry*, 12(2), 144–154.

Helman C (2007) *Culture, Health and Illness*, 5th Edition, Hodder Arnold, London.

Holland C K (1993) An ethnographic study of nursing culture as an exploration for determining the existence of a system of ritual, *Journal of Advanced Nursing*, 18, 1461–1470.

Holland K (1999) A journey to becoming: The student nurse in transition, *Journal of Advanced Nursing*, 29(1), 1461–1470.

Holland K (2017) *Cultural Awareness in Nursing and Health Care. An Introductory Text*, 3rd Edition, Routledge, London.

Jiyane P M, Phiri S S & Peu M D (2012) Nurses' experiences of the ritual of fetching the spirit of the deceased from a public hospital in Mpumalanga, South Africa, *Africa Journal of Nursing and Midwifery*, 14(1), 116–129.

La Fontaine J S (1985) *Initiation: Ritual Drama and Secret Knowledge Across the World*, Penguin Books, Harmondsworth.

Lee D S (2001) The morning tea break ritual: A case study, *International Journal of Nursing Practice*, 7, 69–73.

Loudan J B (1966) Private Stress and Public Ritual, *Journal of Psychosomatic Research*, 10(1), 101–108.

McAllister M (2008) Thank-you cards: Reclaiming a nursing student ritual and releasing its transformative potential, *Nurse Education in Practice*, 8, 170–176.

MacGuire J M (1968) The function of the 'set' in hospital controlled schemes of nurse training, *The British Journal of Sociology*, 19(3), 271–283.

Menzies I E P (1960) A case-study in the functioning of social systems as a defence against anxiety, *Human Relations*, Tavistock Publications, London.

Merton R (1956) Social theory and social structure, Free Press, New York.

Nursing and Midwifery Council (2018) *Future Nurse: Standards of Proficiency for Registered Nurses*, NMC, London.

O'Gorman S M (1998) Death and dying in contemporary society: An evaluation of current attitudes and the rituals associated with death and dying and their relevance to recent understandings of health and healing, *Journal of Advanced Nursing*, 27(6), 1127–1135.

Philpin S M (2002) Rituals and nursing: A critical commentary, *Journal of Advanced Nursing*, 38(2), 144–151.

Philpin S M (2004) *An Interpretation of Ritual and Symbolism in an Intensive Therapy Unit*, Unpublished PhD study, University of Wales Swansea, Swansea.

Philpin S M (2006) 'Handing over': Transmission of information between nurses in an intensive therapy unit, *Nursing in Critical Care*, 11(2), 86–93 (http://ethos.bl.uk/OrderDetails.do?did=1&uin=uk.bl.ethos.606379).

Philpin S M (2007) Managing ambiguity and danger in an intensive therapy unit: ritual practices and sequestration, *Nursing Inquiry*, 14(1), 51–59.

Pountney L & Maric T (2015) *Introducing Anthropology: What Makes us Human?*, 1st Edition, Polity Press, Cambridge.

Schultz E A & LavendaR H (2013) *Cultural Anthropology: A Perspective on the Human Condition*, Oxford University Press, Oxford.

Silberger M R (1998) Tracing our rituals in nursing, *Nursing Leadership Forum*, 3(1), 8–12.

Strange F (2001) The persistence of ritual in nursing practice, *Clinical Effectiveness in Nursing*, 5, 177–183.

Suominen T, Kovasim M & Ketola O (1997) Nursing culture – some viewpoints, *Journal of Advanced Nursing Studies*, 25, 186–190.

Templeman J (2015) *An ethnographic study of critical care nurses' experiences following the decision to withdraw life-sustaining treatment from patients in a UK intensive care unit*, Unpublished PhD study, University of Salford, Salford.

Teres D (1993) Civilian triage in the intensive care unit: The ritual of the last bed, *Critical Care Medicine*, 21(4), 598–606.

Turner V (1969) *The Ritual Process: Structure and Anti-Structure*, Aladine De Gruyter, New York.

Van Gennep A (1960) *The Rites of Passage*, University of Chicago Press, Chicago.

Walker V H (1967) *Nursing and Ritualistic Practice*, Macmillan, New York.

Walsh M & FordP (1989) *New Rituals for Old*, Butterworth Heinemann, Oxford.

Walsh M & FordP (1994) *Nursing Rituals, Research and Rational Actions*, Heinemann Nursing, Oxford.

Wolf Z R (1986a) Nurses' work: The sacred and the profane, *Holistic Nursing Practice*, 1(1), 29–35.

Wolf Z R (1986b) *Nursing Rituals in an Adult Acute Care Hospital: An Ethnography*, Unpublished PhD study, School of Nursing, University of Pennsylvania, Philadelphia.

Wolf Z R (1988a) Nursing rituals, *The Canadian Journal of Nursing Research*, 20(3), 59–69.

Wolf Z R (1988b) *Nurses' Work: The Sacred and the Profane*, University of Pennsylvania, Pennsylvania.

Wolf Z R (1997) Nursing students experience bathing patients for the first time, *Nurse Educator*, 22(2), 41–46.

Wolf Z R (2014) *Exploring Rituals in Nursing: Joining Art and Science*, Springer Publishing Company, New York.

Further reading

1   Brooks I & Macdonald S (2000) 'Doing life': Gender relations in a night nursing sub-culture, *Gender, Work and Organisation*, 7(4), 221–229.

2   Davis-Floyd R E (1987) Obstetric training as a rite of passage, *Medical Anthropology Quarterly*, 1(3), 288–318.

3   Hendry J (2016) *An Introduction to Social Anthropology*, 3rd Edition, Palgrave, London.

4   Hockey J (1990) *Experiences of Death: An Anthropological Account*, Edinburgh University Press, Edinburgh.

5   Shield R R (2015) *Uneasy Endings: Daily Life in an American Nursing Home*, Cornell University Press, Ithaca.

6   Turner V (1982) *From Ritual to Theatre: The Human Seriousness of Play*, PAJ Publications, New York.

7   Winkelman M (2009) *Culture and Health: Applying Medical Anthropology*, Jossey-Bass, San Francisco.

6

TRANSITION AND INITIATION

The student nurse

Karen Holland

Introduction

Student nurses learn to become a nurse through an educational process that ensures their entry into the occupational culture that is nursing, whilst at the same time being able to undertake 'nursing' work and be employed as a nurse in one of many health care settings.

This nursing culture exists within the wider context of an organisational culture such as that of the health care service of the hospital. Rosen (1963) saw the hospital as '*a cornerstone of any modern system of health care*' (p. 1), where looking after the sick was essential in managing illness through creating safe environments '*for personal care and shelter*' as well as offering medical treatments. In today's health care systems this position of the hospital in different societies worldwide has retained its importance as a place to '*learn to become a nurse*', although of course, certainly in the UK, much of the care of patients now takes place in the community. I will be considering these different environments in which health care takes place, as they have become a major challenge for the student nurse's journey or transition experiences, from being known as a student of nursing to becoming an actual qualified nurse.

Student nurse and occupational boundaries

All students are expected to experience the reality of different nursing work environments (known as placements) in order to 'pass through' various stages of their journey to becoming a nurse. Melia (1987) calls this 'transience' and her work is one of the key studies that resonates with my own experience and observations of student nurses learning to become nurses. The other important concept that is seen in the literature in relation to student nurses learning to become a nurse, is that of socialisation, where it is more about how the students learn to undertake their future role, what they have to do to become a member of their new cultural group and how they 'get through' their planned and staged transition. This is a parallel process to the actual stages of an initiation or rites of passage as identified by Van Gennep (1960). I had in fact identified this transition as part of nursing's cultural system, where there were clearly '*arrangements for the socialisation of new members*' (Holland 1993, p. 1462).

The prescribed educational journey, however, also sees the student nurse having to be exposed to the private domain of health care, that is the home. This is only if we are talking about those societies where there is a very clear distinction from the hospital where those who are sick can be housed for their 'safety' or to keep their sickness away from society as a whole. It is where sickness is traditionally contained (see Littlewood 1991).

The ongoing changes to health care where there is evidence of a quicker recovery from serious illness, means that the student has to learn to be able to work across both boundaries; one where there is a blurring of the care needs of the patient who is discharged from a hospital only then to have those care needs managed in the home environment within the community.

The transition to becoming a nurse now encapsulates the two major environments which also challenges the student nurse's socialisation into a nursing culture, which also has its own subcultures within the environment of the hospital; for example, that found in the Intensive Care Unit. The change in care environments has, however, also created additional sub-cultures of nursing in the community settings, such as the environment of the hospice or the prison setting. Both of these, and many others of course, are challenging environments in which some student nurses may find themselves being placed for a learning experience. I will be discussing this part of the student experience in more depth later because I believe that the allocation of a student nurse to specific clinical placements during their transition to becoming a nurse is a critical part of an initiation pathway that each student will undertake as a group, but where each student will follow their own unique pathway.

These experiences, along with others, ensure that the student nurse's initiation into the wider nursing culture is tribal in nature, that is they follow a nomadic pattern of existence in their moving from place to place in order to learn their future role or position in their social and professional group. Their whole journey, their initiation and transition from student to qualified nurse is governed by the rules set down in their curriculum and other professional and legal requirements. This chapter will explore these issues against the premise that student nurses undertake one kind of initiation, albeit that which could be argued by some, in anthropological terms, a metaphorical one. However, in my first exploration of this journey (Holland 1999) the transition of the student nurse to qualified nurse was clearly a rite of passage as well as a status passage although not a clearly defined event, as possibly in the 1960s when I was training, and especially given the changes taking place from external pressures, both societal and political, in health care generally.

It will be important that readers refer to Chapter 5 on rituals in order to engage fully with this chapter, although there will be some overlap of some of the issues as they relate to initiation.

Learning to be a nurse: historical context and models

Nurses inhabit a 'subcultural' world within the predominant culture of the society in which they exist and are a group of individuals drawn together because of the social adversaries of illness and disease. Due to social change the role of nurses has changed from one of altruism and dedication in 'doing good works' to one of a paid occupation (see Chapter 7). Nurses undertake their role within many different environments, with the central location for sick people remaining the hospital.

Learning to nurse or carry out the work of nursing is essential to ensure 'safety' of the sick and also that there are clearly defined stages that are adhered to in order to ensure that the role of nurse (Registered) and indeed the title itself is worthy (in Professional terms and in law) of those that undergo various examinations and what one might call 'tests of endurance' over a set period of time.

The whole experience, from the period before becoming a student nurse (*separation* from prior role as in Van Gennep's work) through their *transition* as a student nurse until they pass various tests to enter their new state as a qualified and registered nurse (*incorporation* – Van Gennep), and they can also be acknowledged as experiencing a period of socialisation into the actual culture of nursing itself (Esterhuizen 2010).

Some readers may argue that I should be looking at these separately through a sociological and an anthropological lens, but as there is significantly more literature on the socialisation of student nurses than viewed from an anthropological perspective, I have chosen to consider some of the major work in this area alongside the latter. Some of course encapsulates both (Melia 1987).

When learning to undertake a new role within the wider society in which they live, individuals can be seen to undergo a period of socialisation and are usually introduced to their intended future role by those who are experienced in that role itself.

In traditional societies, for example, changing role is usually within the province of age and gender, when 'novitiates' as they are called, undergo a transition process which includes a series of initiation rites. In more complex societies such role transitions are infinitely more difficult to visualise in such simplistic social divisions of age and gender, because such societies are also multiple social realities of different cultural groups.

Anthropologists in the past studied what were often called ' primitive ' tribal societies throughout the world, where boundaries were much more easily defined (Mead 1928; Mead 1930). However, today, for varied reasons, such cultural boundaries have become much more blurred and anthropologists have started to study smaller 'subcultures' of the wider social groups, which still retain the idea of a 'tribal society' (Johnson 1987). Nurses are one such group being studied, anthropologically, within bounded areas focused on different smaller specialities in existence, in particular because of defined medical diagnoses of the patient's illness (see Chapter 5). For two excellent examples of such specialities consider the doctorate studies of Philpin (2004) and Seymour (1997) as they relate to Intensive Care Units.

In order to ensure the continuity of traditional cultural knowledge and beliefs required to ensure the continued existence of a cultural group, there usually exists a mode of cultural transference. In what could be called traditional tribal societies this occurs through gender role initiation and age rituals, along with socialisation. In more complex larger societies this transference is entrusted to education, the exact nature of which is directed through what is known as the educational curriculum. This happens at primary and secondary schools in the UK education system, but in terms of this chapter, also in nursing education through a nursing curriculum. McLaren (1999), in his research in a Catholic school in Canada, saw education as a cultural system, with a central element of this as a ritual performance, where traditional values of the Catholic faith were challenged and evolved. He saw 'schooling' as a ritual performance and that culture '*refer to a system of symbols in accordance with the proponents of the "symbolic-system" school of thought exemplified in the work of Victor Turner, Clifford Geertz ... and others*' (p. 5). His work resonates with my own beliefs about culture and ritual as it relates to student nurse transition to becoming qualified nurses (Holland 1999).

Student nurses as a group are dependent on such a model of transference. Kalisch & Kalisch (1987, p. 3) state that:

Nursing, like all other professions, rests on a cultural base – every occupation must exist within some kind of structure, some kind of ordered world. Our culture provides clues about where nurses and nursing fit into the grand scheme of things.

Student nurses learn to become nurses through an ordered educational process that ensures their entry into the occupational culture that is nursing.

White & Ewan (1991) believed that *'the process of becoming a nurse is a social one'* and as such should be differentiated from the *'academic process of earning a degree or qualification'*. They believed that:

> The latter process signifies that the individual has the required attitudes, skills and knowledge to practice competently. In contracts professional socialisation is the process by which the individual learns the culture of nursing: that combination of symbols, custom and shared meaning which makes nursing distinctive (p. 189).

This issue of learning the culture of nursing, as described here, sees that it is something where nurses, regardless of where they practise in their professional role, would immediately understand each other's nursing context and their socialisation experience as a student nurse. This would mean, for example, that they would understand about the historical development of nursing as a profession and in particular who Florence Nightingale was and also, from today's nursing literature, who Mary Seacole was. (See Seacole's autobiographies from 1857 and 1858, edited and introduced by Sara Salih 2005.) Reading the chronology by Salih of Seacole's life it is clear that not only had she lived a very varied life but she had been committed to caring for sick people all her life.

In the UK there is now a statue of Mary Seacole in the grounds of St Thomas's Hospital in London (see the Mary Seacole Trust website: https://www.maryseacoletrust.org.uk/mary-seacole-statue/).

Florence Nightingale in particular has become a major symbol of the nursing profession, as well as the lamp she carries in photos and drawings of her. She is known as the Lady with the Lamp, and is meant to epitomise all that nursing represents; she is now part of the 'folk lore' that surrounds the nursing profession. (See Chapter 5 for reference to the very symbolic annual service in Westminster Abbey.)

Since Miss Nightingale's era the context around the student nurse (known then as a probationer) has had a major influence on their experience. This includes not only the cultural context but also the political and social context in which nursing takes place, as well as the temporal and spatial (see Chapter 4).

Learning to nurse takes place within two parallel settings which Melia (1984) refers to as segments: one, the educational institution, and the other, the (clinical) practice settings where qualified nurses undertake their occupational roles. This dual-role reality ensures that the student exists in what Schmalenberg & Kramer (1979) call a 'bicultural world', and that this 'double existence' created for many graduate nurses a situation called 'reality shock' especially when moving from the educational/school of nursing environment to that of the reality of clinical practice. Others call this pattern of change 'culture shock'.

This dual reality in which student nurses find themselves in has what could be called conflicting ideologies, and the main one has centred on the perceived theory–practice gap thought to exist because of the idealism of educationalists in a university setting and the realism of the practitioners. This is in my view a false argument, in that theory and practice are not synonymous with competing ideologies, namely that theory is distinct from practice and therefore they cannot be derived from each other. It is also seen in the experience of the student nurse who may see that what is often taught in college cannot possibly be experienced in the reality of clinical practice.

In a later study Duchscher (2008) called this moving from one role to another, as well as one place to another, 'transition shock' when it came to student nurses making the change and transition to being a newly qualified graduate nurse. In my study of this transition for student nurses (Holland 1999, p. 232) I discovered that there were '*three states that take place as students undergo the change: becoming a student nurse, being a student nurse and becoming a qualified nurse*'. I related these to Van Gennep's (1960) subdivisions in his rites of passage work: namely separation, transition and incorporation.

Infante (1985) highlights the time lapse between learning and practice, in that students are often assigned to activities in clinical practice before they have learnt the underlying concepts and acquired appropriate skills. One could argue, then, that there will never be a match between learning in university and learning in practice because of time – and also because one cannot predict what students need to know in the clinical environment when they undertake placement learning. I have already considered the uniqueness of nursing, and also every nurse–patient encounter in Chapter 2, which in my view supports the premise that student nurses learning to nurse cannot be taught the theory nor the practice of everything that will be experienced by not only one student in one placement but, in some of the larger groups of students (for example 350), multiple placements and multiple encounters. We can consider these experiences in the next section on the initiation of the student nurse.

Closely linked to the states of transition, as described above, is the experience we know as socialisation and in particular its dual nature, and it is viewed as a means by which an individual as part of society '*absorbs its cultural mores*'. According to Easthope (1980), for the purpose of his explanation, education is '*socialisation carried out with deliberate and planned intent*' within specific socialisation settings. Based on the work of Wheeler (1966) he notes that there are three ideal types of settings:

> where some people are formally charged with the task of influencing others so that they will leave the setting with different skills, attitudes, values and other qualities from those with which they entered (Easthope 1980, p. 154).

This belief (theory) appears to imply that there is a similar spatial and temporal existence to that found within transition states and associated rites, and he identified the three ideal types of settings as:

- Communal resocialisation agencies
- Apprenticeship
- Schooling

These ideal types and their implications as determined by Easthope (1980) have in fact underpinned much of the historical literature on the development of nursing as an occupation and profession. *Apprenticeship* and *Schooling* also correspond to exact periods of time in nursing history, yet they are not mutually exclusive to one another in relation to current practice. We can consider briefly their meaning as they relate to what we know about their relationship to student nurses' transition to becoming a nurse.

1. Communal resocialisation agencies

In this first type, there are three distinguishable elements, namely:

a   Stripping of the old self
b   Denial of an active self
c   Provision of a new self

These stages have a parallel in Van Gennep's rites of passage, where the old self gives way to the new self through a series of events and tests (see Chapter 5). Having considered East-hope's explanation, there are elements of his meaning in the way in which the student nurse enters nursing, progresses through the programme and becomes someone else because of it. The person joins the group of others starting their journey, although there is no major stripping away of the old self as in the kind of 'cloister' behaviour that used to happen in Florence Nightingale's times: students would be living away from the 'outside world' and living in nurses' homes where there were very strict rules on what they were allowed to do; that would have been very different to their home lives. They were 'stripped' of their previous way of life and entered into a much more secular existence as well as an ordered one. Olsen & Whittaker (1968), in their study of the professional socialisation of a small group of students in the USA, referred to this separation into the hospital school with an attached residence *'as having a close resemblance to a convent'* (p. 65). One of the major outcomes from their study was the realisation that student nurses were not 'passive recipients' in their transition but in fact took an active part in their socialisation.

I started nurse training, as it was called then in 1967, much as the students in Olsen and Whittaker's research group in the USA, so I experienced this idea of the 'stripping away of self' process, in particular the moving away from home, which was for me at 18 years of age a huge step, travelling 250 miles away and not knowing anyone, joining the 'set' as described by MacGuire (1968) with its numerical identity (September '67), allocated a room in the nurses' home along with others in my 'set'. These were to be my cultural group for the next three years, each of us from very unique backgrounds but pulled together because of our intention to train to become a nurse. That was and had to become, if you wanted to succeed, our raison d'être – our reason for being there. We were known on the wards by this set number and calendar month for many different purposes, none more so than what we were allowed to do in the ward areas. As first years we had to focus on certain skills and tasks and so on up to third year, and this hierarchical expectation of a student nurse remains still with us today. We all learnt quite quickly, however, what one had to be able to do to survive; not only the actual transition process but also those 'hidden cultural rules' that were not taught in a formal sense but were learnt through engaging with peers and others, including the patients who often helped new nurses learn the routine of daily hospital ward life. One I particularly recall was to cultivate the art of 'looking busy'!

Fealy (2006) describes this very well in *A History of Apprenticeship Nurse Training in Ireland*, where not only was the 'set' a way of gaining friends and companionship during training but he also believed that *'the set had important social and symbolic functions'* and *'had the features and functions of a sub-culture'* (p. 134). He also refers to the work and views of MacGuire (1968) on her consideration of the function of the set in hospitals, which was mainly related to the need to ensure that there was a continual supply of students in the workforce and according to her a *'cheap labour force'* (MacGuire 1968, p. 271). She also saw nursing as a social system with similar relationships to that of a Samoan age–grade structured society which Margaret Mead had described (MacGuire 1968, p. 280), where the 'hospital set' described already clearly demonstrated similar characteristics (see Chapter 5).

Easthope's explanation of the way in which the 'agency' had an impact on the lives of those in such a situation is clearly food for thought in terms of a student nurse today who engages with a new self identity as a student nurse, has to experience certain rules and regulations, undertake many tests of endurance and is socialised into the nursing culture where their initial identity as a non-student nurse changes to take on the new self. This remains until they complete their three-year course of study, where they again undergo another similar experience as a qualified nurse seeking employment in a specific nursing speciality area. At this time, however, we can see that numerical labelling still occurs which gives a qualified nurse an identity which those of the nursing culture will, if working in the UK for example, understand regardless of their place of work; that is, another number or Band number. They become known in employment terms as a Band 5 or a Band 6. Other countries will have similar ways of either naming or labelling nurses, and even in the UK these still exist alongside those of the employment grades and are associated with a certain status in the working environment. Examples you may have come across are: Ward Sister, Ward Manager, Staff Nurse (Junior and Senior), Matron.

2.Apprenticeship

Apprenticeship as a term in the workplace has returned to the nursing language in the UK, with new ways for increasing the health care workforce, and this is also used as a means of entry to becoming a qualified nurse (NHS England: https://www.england.nhs.uk/wp-con tent/uploads/2018/03/apprenticeship-scheme.pdf). However, we will only consider it briefly in the context of another way of becoming part of the overall nursing culture.

Easthope (1980) believes that the difference with the other two types of socialisation settings is merely a matter of 'emphasis' rather than absolute 'divide' and that the achievement of identity change is very much dependent upon the 'one master' with whom the apprentice has a 'strong hierarchical relationship'. Although this has been explored as it relates to the clinical learning environment (Jacka & Lewin 1987), Infante (1985, p. 20) does not believe that all the elements of a true apprenticeship are present in nursing. The use of *'a number of practitioners as role models who may or may not be master practitioners'* make it more akin to *'worker type on the job training experiences'* rather than a true apprenticeship. Jacka & Lewin (1987) highlight two elements in an apprenticeship that for them created some complexity. These were that in an apprenticeship there is an assumption of *'learning by doing and learning by being with an expert'* (p. 29). For a student nurse both these are important when learning in the clinical learning environment and are interlinked. However, as we have seen, their journey takes place in two main environments, which includes the university setting where they are a student involved in 'academic' study, alongside their placements to learn their future occupational role by actually 'learning by doing' nursing.

This type of socialisation is at present confusing the traditional transition from student nurse to qualified nurse, with a number of new pathways to either the main pathway of becoming a student nurse (as with the Nursing Apprenticeship) or joining in at a later stage of the journey through the acquisition of certain skills and knowledge. In fact I found the beginning of a confused pattern in the study of the transition of the student nurse to become a qualified nurse (Holland 1999), as I also found the dual roles that many student nurses had already, by working as a health care assistant alongside being a student, the main reason for this being to earn money to add to their student funding. However, this dual role created for me two main questions which are important to any transition or initiation into their future role:

> First if students are undertaking both roles simultaneously, when and how do they learn to internalise their future professional/occupational role culture and its associated accountability? Second, who is teaching them the skills required of a registered nurse in relation to essential care-giving when it is apparent that if a student works as a health care assistant in one role, they are deemed competent to be undertaking these same skills as a student nurse? (Holland 1999, p. 233.)

This dual role is ongoing today, from conversations with student nurses during my 'service user' role in the outpatient departments of local hospitals, after they have introduced themselves to me. It is also evident that those I have met are very aware of the role that they are undertaking when employed as a health worker and are not there to learn as a student nurse.

The nursing shift from a stronger apprenticeship-type model of learning to become a nurse to what we have now has been evident through the various changes in nursing education in the UK and indeed elsewhere. This is as a nursing student, being educated in the 'subject of nursing' in a university setting (with its own transition rites) alongside learning to undertake aspects of their future work and role alongside their peers and under the guidance and teaching of their 'experienced and qualified' role models (multiple 'masters' with different skills/knowledge sets dependent on the environment in which they are working) plus a whole range of other health professionals. That is, everyone who is involved in health care delivery can now be involved in the learning experience of the student nurse – thus changing completely the idea of the wholly apprenticeship-type model. Not only that but in terms of the actual individual who has deliberately sought to enter into a transition from student nurse to qualified nurse, there are now multiple routes to this end. This is problematic, however, from what we are considering in this chapter about the idea of a transition or initiation into the nursing culture and finally being that registered qualified nurse and what it means in society at large, is that like many traditional cultures that have been subject to major change to their boundaries and their way of life, nursing as a cultural group may well be at this cross-roads where those initial boundaries around its professional role and existence need to be restored again. This is another topic beyond the scope of this chapter but I will be returning to this in Chapter 7.

3. Schooling

Schooling, in contrast to the other settings, has two distinct features, that is separation of education from work and ordering of the education process. As in the rites associated with transition and status passage there is an implied separation from a prior state of existence, in this instance that of the physical separation of that being learnt from the place where it 'actually exists in reality', i.e. the separation of the nursing school from the clinical workplace in the case of nursing. We saw this initially with the shift of schools of nursing away from the hospitals where the students were situated, and although there were major political and economic reasons for this shift, there had also been a recognition through a variety of working groups and evaluation of nursing as a developing profession (UKCC 1987). McLaren (1999) offers us a unqiue way of considering schooling – which he deems as a 'ritual performance'. He makes the point that:

> it is educationally important to recognise and understand the cultural politics of ritual performance. Because rituals transmit societal and cultural ideologies, we can discover a lot about 'how ideologies do their work' by examining key symbols and root paradigms of the ritual system of the school (p. xiii).

In this chapter we will explore next what we can learn about the nature of a 'ritual performance' that the student nurse experiences in the transition from one state of being to another. I will not, however, be able to undertake a detailed examination of this in relation to the history of nursing over a long period of time. Instead I will describe from my own observations and experience, supported by various forms of evidence as well as the initial assumption I have already made in this book, that nursing is a culture and would therefore have a system of ritual through which members of one generation 'pass on' its traditional knowledge etc. via a ritual performance of an initiation (see Chapter 2.)

Learning to nurse: place and time

In order to become a registered nurse and given the power that comes with this role in relation to patient care, patient safety and treatment of vulnerable groups in society, nurses are required to undergo a period of 'training and education' over a prescribed period of time. This is normally three years (although there are variations as change in health care and the nursing workforce demands), where students gain practical learning in their future workplace, caring for patients and families, under the supervision and guidance, as well as assessment and surveillance, of registered nurses and qualified others. In addition students are taught in a university setting and gain clinical experience in a simulated learning laboratory, gaining knowledge and skills which are perceived as being necessary for them being able to undertake the role of a qualified nurse in employment at the end of their three-year transition.

This separation, one can argue, has created a separation of 'know-how knowledge' (that is practical knowledge of doing nursing and the skills to perform nursing activities) from 'know that knowledge' (theoretical knowledge of how nursing should be carried out and the kind of knowledge required to undertake it or its performance in practice). One of the outcomes of the major change to nursing and nurse education which became known as Project 2000 in the UK (UKCC 1986) was described by Slevin (1992) as 'Knowledgeable doing' (p. 26) and a term to which the student nurses undergoing this new way of educating and training nurses were then known as was 'the knowledgeable doer' (p. 27). There were, as with any change, many differing views on the future of nursing, and in fact on reflection it was not unlike the difference of opinion between Florence Nightingale and Mrs Bedford Fenwick (see Chapter

2). The result in both changes was a major shift in how future (registered) nurses were to be educated and trained for their role. In both cases a cultural shift took place in what this transition was to look like.

According to Abel-Smith (1960, p.62) Mrs Bedford Fenwick saw nurse training as:

> an apprenticeship, a period of trial, almost an initiation ritual, to test who was fit to bear the title nurse. The greater its severity the higher its intellectual demands, the longer its duration, the greater the status of the professional. The very fact that every woman thought she could nurse made it more necessary to emphasise and exaggerate training requirements.

The objective of the initiation is to prepare the student to take on the role of a qualified nurse who undertakes nursing work (see Chapter 7); to be a nurse and do nursing work.

In preparation for this they are also expected to pursue other learning to gain an academic qualification as well as a professional one, which demonstrates their employability in what we can call the 'market place'. This is through having a higher-education qualification as evidence of skills and knowledge which are intended to make them more employable as a nurse but also the recognition that nursing as a career has credibility in the wider employment market. This pursuit of higher intellectual capabilities, whilst retaining that caring image of the nurse in relation to sick people, has in many ways created tensions for what should be retained as 'belonging' to the title nurse, and what indeed can easily be part of another role without the attendant expected level of knowledge and skills for the future that is required of a qualified and registered nurse. This title is protected in law, in much the same way as a registered (medical) doctor is. (See how these and other health professionals' titles are protected by law in the UK as part of the wider patient and public safety regulations: https://www.professionalstandards. org.uk/docs/default-source/publications/policy-advice/tackling-misuse-of-protected-ti tle-2010.pdf?sfvrsn=d8c77f20_10.) Anyone using the title of nurse in a role that clearly demands that they are registered to do so, without their being recorded as having this right, is doing so illegally and putting patients at risk (The Council for Healthcare Regulatory Excellence 2010). Obtaining registration as a nurse is associated with being given a unique number, and became a part of nursing culture that has existed since the Register was started in September 1921.

Initiation of student nurse: temporal, spatial and cultural context

We can see in Box 6.1 all the aspects of an initiation as defined by La Fontaine (see Chapter 5 for more detail) and I will use these headings to demonstrate how the student nurse journey to becoming a qualified nurse (Holland 1999) contains all of these steps in one form or another. However, it is also very important that we consider this initiation or rites of passage for the student nurse in what are clearly three very important contexts which have been discussed already in previous chapters (see Chapter 5). A doctor's initiation into medicine culture interestingly follows a similar historical pathway and pattern to that of nursing (Konner 1987; Sinclair 1997; Bucher & Stelling 1977).

BOX 6.1 ASPECTS OF AN INITIATION (AS DEFINED BY LA FONTAINE 1985)

1. Social action
2. Rules of participation
3. Rules of exclusion
4. General recognition of correct pattern of what should be followed
5. Has a fixed structure and is prescriptive, i.e. it must be done
6. Tests and ordeals
7. Oaths and affirmations

The student initiation is governed by time, space and culture, as is nursing work itself (see Chapter 4), and is clearly nomadic as can be seen in the student nurses' patterns of learning over their three-year course of study and practice to become a nurse. This pattern is made of various periods of learning in clinical practice or clinical placements, which are a number of bounded experiences which are inter-linked with the illness experiences of the patients (see Box 6.2).

BOX 6.2 EXAMPLES OF BOUNDED PLACEMENT EXPERIENCES FOR STUDENT NURSES

1. Surgical ward
2. Medical ward
3. Orthopaedic ward
4. Operating theatres
5. Forensic mental health ward
6. Child and adolescent mental health
7. Children's Intensive Care Unit
8. Community Health Centre*
9. Dermatology Outpatients
10. University setting*

   *The * placements are not 'patient-related' specific and 10 is actually their base placement where they return to between each of the other clinical placements*

The following description of aspects of an initiation is based on unpublished post-graduate work which had ethical approval and successful examination of the research proposal, as well as some early data analysis and findings. Student approval was also given for sharing their narratives and the findings. It is also based in part on previous ethnographic research undertaken for Master's-level study (Holland 1999).

The placement as a context for initiation

Students' whole period of initiation and transition to becoming a nurse is built into these bounded units of experiences (Spaces), including that one main 'placement' in the university setting, although even in this setting we can now see the increasing importance of two different placement types: that of the actual physical classroom (Space) where learning is experienced, but also the increasing reliance on the clinical simulation laboratory (Space) for the learning of clinical skills and knowledge instead of or in preparation for their clinical placement experience. (This experience is controlled in terms of time by the nurses' professional body, the Nursing and Midwifery Council.)

Although student nurses will begin their 'nomadic' journey together as a group with a number of others, their pathways will initially differ according to their eventual workplace employment field. These are known respectively as Adult Nursing, Children's Nursing, Mental Health Nursing and Learning Disability Nursing fields of practice. In fact if we were to consider in detail each of these fields in their broadest sense we can see that in fact they can be considered major subcultures within the overarching nursing culture, with each being able to show further delineation into further smaller subcultures such as Coronary Heart Care, Surgical Nursing (Holland & Roxburgh 2012), Paediatric Oncology or Forensic Mental Health (see Chapter 2).

Secondly, again depending on their chosen field of practice, students will be required to undertake certain placements (as a pattern to their nomadic life journey) during their course of study in the university and practice learning environments in order to achieve certain rules and regulations laid down by the professional body of the NMC. In addition, and key to their successful initiation and passage to becoming a qualified nurse, is what I call the cultural 'rule book' which is the validated curriculum which as we have seen previously offers a 'blueprint' for their initiation process and is similar to the fixed structure and prescriptive characteristics of an initiation stage (see Box 6.1).

Regardless of their communal beginning as a group, however, each participant in this journey will have a unique experience through their initiation/transition, even with an overarching circumscribed curriculum for the essentials of what they have to be taught. This is seen more in the relation to their clinical placement pathways because when in the university placement setting (Space) they have to pursue similar experiences and are taught specific content that is prescribed by the curriculum. For example, learning how to give an injection is a skill that can be required in any field of nursing practice and is one of those 'initiation rites' which has to be undertaken and successfully achieved at some point in their three-year initiation, if only to have completed what many student nurses fear they will be unable to undertake. One could argue that for many this is due to the fear of harming the patient which remains inbuilt into their learning to be a 'good nurse' who does no harm. (I will not enter into any detailed discussion and specific nuances here to the overarching curriculum requirements – simply because it would take me on a tangent beyond the specific aims of the chapter.)

There are specific cultural and written rules as to who should participate in the students' learning, in particular in relation to how they are tested to become a qualified nurse. In the practice environment this will be the clinical assessor and in the university the academic assessor (Nursing and Midwifery Council 2018a). These will be accorded official roles in their initiation and given the power and rights to pass or fail students. This issue of not failing students has been a long-standing challenge for nursing mentors and assessors, who could be referred to as the senior members of the 'nursing tribe'.

In terms of oaths and affirmations all students are expected to uphold a professional Code of Conduct (in the UK this is known as: The Code 2018 – Nursing and Midwifery Council

2018b) as student nurses and agree to abide by a set of Standards for aspects of practice – with an overarching principle of 'doing the patient no harm'. On qualifying as a student nurse they are then registered as nurses and they accept accountability for actions in relation to their nursing work. They are 'tested' to take on this role at various intervals during their three years to determine their 'fitness for practice' (Nursing and Midwifery Council 2018a) This relates to various tests in both practice fields and in the University setting as both their professional and academic awards are interlinked in their transition.

Temporality and the initiation

Every initiation has a temporal context and gives it form (see Chapter 5). It has a fixed structure and this is prescriptive (La Fontaine 1985). Regardless of where this takes place in the UK there is an overarching fixed structure laid down in Statute (Nurses, Midwives and Health Visitors' Approval Order 1989) and consists of three distinct years with expectations of successful attainment of achievement at certain periods during these three years. The curriculum maps out this length of time into other distinct periods of time known as 'modules', which are to be found within other separate bounded units known as Nursing Semesters, which are again of varying lengths and both modules and Semesters are counted in a number of weeks. There are other weeks of allocated time for leisure time or holidays as an essential aspect of university life for students. Nursing students, however, are not able to have the same number of holidays because their programme is governed at present by a European Nursing Directive (77/453/EEC Nursing Directive) which controls the overarching number of hours that a nursing programme validated by their professional body the NMC has to have. This is three years or 4,600 hours, divided into 2,300 hours of theory and 2,300 hours of practice. This pattern of hours and weeks and years governs the initiation length and organisation which will also include tests of fitness to practice and various stages. This is important in relation to considering the nurses' journey over three years as an initiation rite, because there are clearly similarities with the rules governing length of time for many initiation rites recorded in tribal cultures, for example.

Time also shapes their experience in practice as these students note:

> It was 6.55am and I was just about to sit down in the office and wait for report before starting the early shift at 7.15am (Adult Nursing field student: 3rd Year).
>
> Being in the middle of the night there were only three nurses and myself a student nurse on duty (Adult Nursing field student: 3rd Year).

We can see here images of Zerubavel (1979) in how time governs actions in a hospital ward. So not only are students expected to undertake their initiation and transition in a specific time, they are then also made to fit in with the time schedule within various placements of learning (see Chapter 4 on Temporality).

Spatiality and the initiation

The context around the student nurse has a major influence on their learning experience and therefore their initiation. We have seen that according to Melia (1984) learning to nurse takes place in two parallel settings she calls segments. This dual reality ensures, however, that the nursing student exists in a bicultural world (Kramer & Schmalenberg 1977) with potentially conflicting ideologies. The main difficulty has centred on the perceived theory and practice gap thought to exist because of the idealism of the educationalists and the realism of the practitioners. This is, however, a false argument in that theory and practice are not synonymous with competing ideologies, namely that theory is distinct from practice and cannot be derived from each other. (See Chapter 4 for more discussion on spatiality.)

Each of the fixed time periods in the curriculum has a virtual boundary, separating out practice time, university time and leisure time. In terms of practice placement time which included a number of wards, not only was time identified but also the physical space where students are expected to undertake their clinical learning. These spaces where student nurses experience nursing work are known as clinical placements and in the hospital space this was further divided into further virtually, and in many cases physically, bounded spaces known as wards. Each ward area also has certain spatial structures, some left over from Nightingale's era with the type of ward named after her – The Nightingale Ward – which are long wards with beds on each side and where the patients can easily be kept under surveillance. (See Chapter 4 and this website for an example and also a number of other historical archives: http://www.kingscollections.org/exhibitions/specialcollections/nightingale-and-hospital-design/florence-nightingale-and-hospital-design.)

Cultural context and the initiation

Initiation takes place within a cultural context and is a social action (La Fontaine 1985). Its main purpose is to initiate the nursing student into nursing work and its culture (see Chapter 7). In terms of the structure and organisation of the initiation, the curriculum can be viewed as the 'symbolic rule book' for what has to happen. However, there is also something that the student nurse has to learn about quite quickly if they are to manage to traverse the tests and engage with the learning experience in both settings of the initiation. This is known as the 'Hidden Curriculum' (Glen 1991) and is as important to a successful transition from student nurse to qualified nurse as is the acknowledged 'seen curriculum'. Despite the unpredictability and uncertainty of their individual initiation experiences, with possible 'culture shock' taking place, it doesn't just happen; that is, it is a planned event in so far as the boundaries of their placement goes. In terms of unpredictable here I mean that it is not possible to predict what kind of individual experience each student nurse has in advance of entering the cultural environment of each placement, including that of the university setting. Only in the latter there is more predictability because of the space involved and what takes place there can be guaranteed in terms of getting taught, gaining instruction and sharing the space with peers and their lecturers.

My study on transition of the student nurses had found three major phases: becoming a student nurse, being a student nurse and becoming a qualified nurse (Holland 1999) so I had already undertaken research that had arrived at a certain level of information and confirmation in many ways of what I have tried to convey here.

What I had discovered from all my fieldwork, analysis of data and later discussion with students was the centrality of the patients to their learning to become nurses. Students talked about 'my patient' and 'handing over' a patient to another nurse – an implicit kind of exchange system, whereby the patients in a ward were handed over during cultural and temporal situations of the ritual of the Handover Report (Holland 1999). I have already begun to pursue more evidence concerning this notion of ownership of both a patient and of one another. It is a field I think for future nursing research.

On a parallel route student nurses themselves were also handed over or passed on from mentor to mentor and assessor to assessor. It is clear that the patient is an 'object' of learning, as they are central not only to nursing work but also as someone that students have to learn from doing things to them, that is they are used as 'tools for learning' – which is an unusual way of thinking about any patient in relation to the student nurse. Here are a few examples:

> *David was allocated to my team as the staff nurse thought it would be an invaluable learning situation* (Children's Nursing student nurse).
>
> *As catheterisation was one of my learning outcomes, my assessor on the ward suggested it would be a good learning experience for me to catheterise Edith* (Student Adult Nursing Field).

In considering the learning experience for the student nurse one can say that it is, over the three years, a fairly hit-and-miss experience given the lack of control on the nature of each clinical placement at least. During their initiation the student nurse can be seen to be very vulnerable in terms of what she/he can achieve to be successful in making that transition to being a qualified nurse. They are dependent not only on the patients themselves, but also the place where they undertake their learning, but most importantly much of their day-to-day learning is in the gift of others, such as their mentors and assessors. We hear of instances where students have not had a good learning experience because of such actions. Learning to fit in is a clear example of what they believe they have to do to 'get through' a placement (Melia 1984). This view of the fact that the student nurse learning and experience of nursing work and patient care is in fact dependent on contact and communication as a kind of 'gift' from the patient or their mentors, especially in relation to the fact that to become a nurse the student is very dependent to some extent on the patient 'gifting' themselves for them to learn, is very much another aspect of their experience that we cannot predict. What do they then receive in return or is there no reciprocity? One can assume, given the situations that nursing takes place in, that as a possible 'gift exchange', the patient receives the 'gift' of care by the student nurse and knowing that they are contributing to their learning. Attending various hospital outpatient departments I have often been invited to explain my 'health condition' to a student nurse and especially how it impacts on my life in general. As a person this makes me feel that someone values my experience as a person, and as an educator twice valued in being able to contribute to the student's learning. Reading a very insightful paper by Adams & Sharp (2013) entitled *Reciprocity in Caring Labor: Nurses' Work in Residential Aged Care in Australia*, based on their own research, I was particularly drawn to their discussion on what they termed 'professional reciprocity' as a way of seeking an answer to my own experience as related to this shared student nurse–patient learning experience. Although their analysis of the literature on reciprocity referred mainly to the nurse–patient relationship in terms of care experiences, I would like to consider that the student nurse learning to become a nurse journey would also be full of reciprocal exchanges. To become a registered qualified nurse the student is dependent on not only engaging with their mentors, who are akin to gatekeepers to their learning experiences with caring for patients, but to those whom they care for. Communication and building relationships with patients and others is a fundamental part of learning to be a nurse. Adams & Sharp (2013) noted that for '*reciprocity to occur, the patient/resident/client must respond and participate in a partnership involving the caregiver and the care recipient*' (p. 10) and in the context of my 'mutual exchanges' with student nurses as a patient (and 'hidden' educator) I was particularly drawn to their explanation about length of time that such reciprocal engagement can happen:

> Further, it has been theorized in the nursing literature that interactions between the nurse and patient are reciprocal to the extent that a 'reciprocal spiral' develops in which these individuals continue to interact or withdraw from the situation. What results is a mutuality or interdependence in which both achieve goals (King 1981, p. 84) (p. 10).

If we consider these views on reciprocity, we can begin to see how important this exchange of communication and care as both learning to become a nurse and learning to care for patients as part of nursing work is during their whole three-year initiation. Also how it becomes an essential issue for those involved in planning specific bounded experiences as placements for the student, plus how they can be supported in practice to engage with a patient so that this can engender a sense of belonging to the nursing community.

Conclusion

Learning to become a nurse takes place, as we have seen, in two major settings which student nurses then have the opportunity to engage in those aspects of nursing practice that they have to learn to either undertake as a skill or learn about in relation to the knowledge required to both practice these skills and to deliver nursing care that is underpinned by a strong evidence base. The continuation of a nursing culture and the inheritance of the traditional cultural knowledge that is part of nursing's inheritance is an essential part of the student nurse transition to becoming a qualified nurse. Within this learning is the essential recognition of the centrality of the patient and also the centrality of the qualified nurses who take on the role of both guide and assessor to determine whether each student nurse does in fact 'pass the test' of joining their new cultural group. They are joined in this endeavour by the collaboration of the two segments in nursing education and practice who plan and approve the broad curriculum as the initiation guide for each future generation of student nurses.

References

Abel-Smith B (1960) *History of the Nursing Profession*, Heinemann Educational Publishers, London.
Adams V & Sharp R (2013) Reciprocity in caring labor: Nurses' work in residential aged care in Australia, *Feminist Economics*, 19(2), 100–121 (http://www2.curtin.edu.au/research/crae/local/docs/9._Reciprocity_in_caring_labor_Published.pdf, accessed 7 July 2019).
Bucher R & Stelling J G (1977) Becoming professional, *The ANNALS of the American Academy of Political and Social Science*, 46, Sage Library of Social Research, Sage Publications, Beverley Hills.
Duchscher J E B (2008) Transition shock: The initial stage of role adaptation for newly graduated registered nurses, *Journal of Advanced Nursing*, 65(6), 1103–1113.
Easthope G (1980) Curricula are social processes. In L Barton, R Meighan & S Walker (1980), *Schooling Ideology and the Curriculum*, 153–168, The Falmer Press, Basingstoke.
Esterhuizen P (2010) *The Journey from Neophyte to Registered Nurse: A Dutch Experience of Professional Socialisation*, VDM Verlag, Germany.
Fealy G (2006) *A History of Apprenticeship Nurse Training In Ireland*, Routledge, London.

Glen S (1991) Planning the ethics component of a curriculum. In S Pendleton & A Myles (eds), *Curriculum Planning in Nursing Education*, Chapter 2, 58–89, Edward Arnold, London.

Holland C K (1993) An ethnographic study of nursing culture as an exploration for determining the existence of a system of ritual, *Journal of Advanced Nursing*, 18, 1461–1470.

Holland K (1999) A journey to becoming: The student nurse in transition, *Journal of Advanced Nursing*, 29(1), 1461–1470.

HollandK & Roxburgh M (2012) *Placement Learning in Surgical Nursing*, Bailliere Tindall, Elsevier, Edinburgh.

Infante M S (1985) *The Clinical Laboratory in Nursing Education*, 2nd Edition, John Wiley & Sons, New York. Originally published in 1975.

Jacka K & Lewin D (1987) *The Clinical Learning of Student Nurses*, King's College London, London.

Johnson M (1997) *Nursing Power and Social Judgement*, Ashgate Publishing, Aldershot.

Kalisch P A & Kalisch B J (1987) *The Changing Image of the Nurse*, Addison Wesley, Menlo Park, California.

King I M (1981) *A Theory for Nursing*, John Wiley & Sons, New York. Cited in V Adams & R Sharp (2013) Reciprocity in caring labor: Nurses' work in residential aged care in Australia, *Feminist Economics*, 19(2), 100–121 (http://www2.curtin.edu.au/research/crae/local/docs/9._Reciprocity_in_caring_labor_Published.pdf, accessed 7 July 2019).

Konner M (1987) *Becoming a Doctor: A Journey of Initiation in Medical School*, Penguin Books, New York.

Kramer M & Schmalenberg C (1977) *Path to Biculturalism*, Contemporary Publishing, Wakefield, Massachusetts.

La Fontaine J S (1985) *Initiation: Ritual Drama and Secret Knowledge Across the World*, Penguin Books, Harmondsworth.

Littlewood J (1991) Care and ambiguity: Towards a concept of nursing. In P Holden & J Littlewood (1991) *Anthropology and Nursing*, Chapter 10, 170–189, Routledge, London.

MacGuire G (1968) The functioning of the 'set' in hospital controlled schemes of nurse training, *British Journal of Sociology*, 19(3), 271–283.

McLaren P (1999) *Schooling as a Ritual Performance: Toward a Political Economy of Educational Symbols and Gestures*, 3rd Edition, Rowan & Littlefield Publishers, Lanham, Maryland.

Mead M (1928) *Coming of Age in Samoa*. Republished in 2001 by Harper Perennial, New York.

Mead M (1930) *Growing Up in New Guinea*, Blue Ribbon Books, New York.

Melia K (1984) Student nurses' construction of occupational socialisation, *Sociology of Health and Illness*, 6(2), 132–151.

Melia K (1987) *Learning and Working: The Occupational Socialisation of Nurses*, Tavistock Publications, London.

Nursing and Midwifery Council (2018a) *Future Nurse: Standards of Proficiency for Registered Nurses*, NMC, London.

Nursing and Midwifery Council (2018b) *The Code: Professional Standards of Practice and Behaviour for Nurses, Midwives and Nursing Associates*, NMC, London.

Nurses, Midwives and Health Visitors (Registered Fever Nurses Amendment Rules and Training Amendment Rules) Approval Order (1989) *The Nurses, Midwives and Health Vistors Act 1979*, UK Government, London (http://www.legislation.gov.uk/uksi/1989/1456/made).

Olsen V L & Whittaker E W (1968) *The Silent Dialogue*, Jossey-Bass, San Francisco.

Philpin S M (2004) *An Interpretation of Ritual and Symbolism in an Intensive Therapy Unit*, Unpublished PhD study, University of Wales Swansea, Swansea.

Rosen G (1963) The hospital: Historical sociology of a community institution. In FriedsonE (ed) *The Hospital in Modern Society*, Chapter 1, 1–36, Collier, London.

Salih S (2005) Introduction. In M Seacole, *Wonderful Adventures of Mrs Seacole in Many Lands*, Penguin Classics, London.

Schmalenberg C & Kramer M (1979), *Coping with Reality Shock: The Voices of Experience*, Nursing Resources, Wakefield.

Seymour J (1997) *Caring for Critically Ill People: A Study in Death and Dying in Intensive Care*, Unpublished PhD study, University of Sheffield, Sheffield.

Sinclair S (1997) *Making Doctors: An Institutional Apprenticeship*, Bloomsbury, London.

Slevin (1992) Knowledgeable doing: The theoretical basis for practice. In O Slevin & M Buckenham *Project 2000: The Teachers Speak*, Chapter 2, 26–41. Campion Press, Edinburgh.

United Kingdom Central Council for Nursing Midwifery and Health Visiting (1987) *Nursing, midwifery and health visiting: A strategy for the reform of education and training*, January, UKCC, London.

UKCC (1986) *Project 2000: A New Preparation for Practice*, UKCC, London.

Van Gennep A (1960) *The Rites of Passage*, Routledge & Kegan Paul, London.

Wheeler S (1966) The structure of formally organised socialisation settings. In BrimO G & WheelerS (eds), *Socialisation of Childhood*, Wiley, New York.

White R & Ewan C E (1991) *Clinical Teaching in Nursing*, Chapman and Hall, London.

Zerubavel E (1979) *Patterns of Time in Hospital Life: A Sociological Perspective*, University of Chicago Press, Chicago.

Further reading

1 Benner O and Benner R V (1979), *The New Nurse's Work Entry: A Troubled Sponsorship*, The Tiresias Press, New York.

2 Glaser B G & Strauss A L (1971) *Status Passage*, Aldine Transaction, New Brunswick.

3 Hamel E J (1990) *An Interpretive Study of the Professional Socialisation (of neophyte nurses into the nursing subculture)*, Dissertation, School of Education, University of San Diego.

4 Mauss M (1954), *The Gift: Forms and Functions of Exchange in Archaic Societies*, Free Press of Glencoe, Illinois. Published in 2011 by Martino Publishing, CT.

5 Morse J M (1989) Gift-giving in the patient-nurse relationship: Reciprocity for care?, *The Canadian Journal of Nursing Research*, 21(1), 33–46.

6 Myers L C (1982) *The Socialisation of Neophyte Nurses*, UMI Research Press, Ann Arbor, Michigan.

7 Pomeranz R (1973) *The Lady Apprentices*, G Bell & Sons, London.

8 Reverby S M (1987) *Ordered to Care: The Dilemma of American Nursing 1859–1945*, Cambridge University Press, Cambridge.

9 Seymour J (2001) *Critical Moments: Death and Dying in Intensive Care*, Open University Press, Milton Keynes.

7

NURSING WORK WITHIN NURSING CULTURE

Images and reality

Karen Holland

Introduction

The purpose and form of nursing work has long been an issue of debate, not just from a philosophical stance but also from an occupational one. The influence for example of the social and political agenda on the scope of nursing work over time has meant that nurses have had to change their practice in order to survive. This need for survival is a global issue, not just as a profession but also as work. In order to explore some of these issues we have already seen that despite change, the culture of nursing retains a common value system and an historical foundation from which it stems.

The nature of nursing work I contend is such an eclectic mixture of skills and knowledge that it is impossible to describe it in a simplistic way, although as we have seen (Chapter 2) many nurse theorists such as Virginia Henderson have tried to do this. Her definition of nursing is one that remains, despite attempts by others to try and define what it is that nurses 'do', what their 'job' is (see Chapter 6).

One can argue that this ambiguity has ensured that it is an easy target for other health care workers and indeed those who employ them, giving the reducing number of nurses in the workforce, to take from nurses the work that has traditionally been seen as nursing. Like all work, nursing can be broken down into distinct tasks or skills in such a way that nurses integrate it into a different context every time they meet a different patient. Nursing work therefore is unique in that sense, in that each nurse–patient relationship is unique (not in form but possibly content), each encounter bringing with it a need to undertake nursing work in an individualised way. Given that nursing is this 'unique blend' I have likened to a kaleidoscope effect – unique at each turn of the nurse–patient contact in a different temporal, spatial and cultural context.

This chapter intends to focus on the actual nature of nursing work, what they are seen to undertake and how this fits in with the overall culture that we can see as nursing. It is not about focusing per se on the actual practice of nursing but on how we can understand how nursing work defines it as a cultural concept, much in the same way that cultures can be seen to have a focus to their daily lives that is unique to them or other related tribal societies: the way in which the Maasai and Samburu tribes in Kenya, for example, revere their cattle which are the source of all their food as well as the focus to their daily 'working' lives, with their care being deeply embedded into their culture and their rituals, including ensuring that they live a very nomadic life in order to ensure their survival. We have been able to see this through ethnographies, books about their culture and for some of us an experience to visit and talk to women and some men in a Maasai village; a glimpse only into their traditional way of life but enough to understand ethnographies of their world by anthropologists and others who lived with them for a longer period of time. (See Ernastina Coast 2000, *Maasai Demography*; an ethnographic study of the Maasai people https://core.ac.uk/download/pdf/ 92476.pdf.)

Nursing work it could be argued has the same sustaining focus, as the wider nursing culture is dependent on it retaining a similar core that can be recognized as the work that sustains nurses in different 'tribal' subcultures. Nurses worldwide can recognize its form and content, through visual images of nurses and nurses at work, reading nursing textbooks or engaging with actual clinical practice.

There is an implicit understanding, for example, that nurses care for patients who are ill (in a hospital or at home) and require care that relies on their unique knowledge and skills or most importantly how these are put together to create the 'care' work that only trained and educated nurses can undertake. This unique blending of nursing work cannot in my view be undertaken by any other health care worker other than a (registered) nurse, whose very existence is supported by their acknowledgement by the nursing 'tribal elders' and their professional laws, namely that of being allowed to call themselves a nurse by virtue of their registering and having passed all the necessary 'tribal tests' to be allowed entry into their next social group in the nursing culture, a qualified registered nurse.

There may well be elements of their cultural knowledge seen in other related health care groups, and it is here where many debates have occurred about the actual reality of what is nursing work, and whether other health care workers can undertake this work. This is not a new situation given the presence of nursing auxiliaries, and it wasn't even when I was training to be a registered nurse in the late 1960s, as they undertook the fundamental care of patients alongside their nursing colleagues. These two roles, as well as another registered nursing role at the same time, that of the Enrolled Nurse (or second-level registered nurse), did register concerns regarding what work they could safely undertake instead of the registered nurse. The Enrolled Nurse role involved two years of training (in the UK) and a focus more on (what I will call for the sake of explaining the difference to those with no nursing background) the more patient-focused practical aspects of nursing work rather than the additional leadership and management work essential for the registered nurse at the time. This role, however, was underpinned by two years of training that involved learning about many of the same subjects and content as the registered nurse pathway, including learning in the same 'bounded' placements experienced by the student nurse. Interestingly the learner enrolled nurse was given their own title – that of the pupil nurse. (See Seccombe et al.'s (1997) *Enrolled Nurses: A Study for the UKCC* which offers an insightful evaluation of the background of the role as well as reasons for its demise in the UK.) The introduction and presence of this role within the nursing culture did impact of course on the initiation dynamics for the student nurses but not such to influence the final transition expectations as a registered nurse. It is beyond the scope of this chapter unfortunately to undertake more than this cursory insight but the Seccombe et al. (1997) study will certainly offer background reading into the role and some of the ongoing debates at the time.

However, the accountability for the overall patient care and indeed safety of that care has remained with the qualified registered nurse responsible for the patient. Other health care workers may undertake what were higher-level skills seen as part of the nurse's work in the past, but the difference is how being registered and named as a nurse 'knits together' the knowledge and skills to make decisions that are beyond the legal responsibility of other health care workers (see Chapter 6). The fact that the UK Nursing and Midwifery Council (2018) has now begun the registration of the new nursing associate in England (see: https://hansard.parliament.uk/pdf/.../2018.../7d84548a-dcdb-460f-940f-fb7729ddf5ec), a role developed to ensure sufficient trained health care workers to support the registered nurse, has of course created much debate about the necessity and potential confusion by the public and service users (see: https://councilofdeans.org.uk/wp-content/uploads/2019/02/031018-CoDH-Scotland-NA-discussion-paper-JN.pdf for some of the debate issues) and of course a return to that old question for nurses – why did we get rid of the Enrolled Nurse role in the UK? (See above reference.)

Before we become diverted into considering these major issues about the nature of nursing work and indeed who 'owns' this in terms of their core values and responsibilities, we need to ensure that we understand what work is in relation to the wider context as well as in relation to nursing. Another term related to work is that of labour and this is an important facet of nursing as can be seen, for example, when discussing the view of nursing as emotional labour (Smith 1992).

Work and labour

Prior to examining the complexity of nursing work it is pertinent to explore the actual meaning of the term 'work'. Grint (1991) argues 'that no unambigious or objective definition of work is possible' and states that:

> Work tends to be an activity that transformed nature and is usually undertaken in social situations, but exactly what counts as work is dependent in the specific social circumstances under which activities are undertaken and, critically, how these circumstances and activities are interpreted by those involved. Whether any particular activity is experienced as work or leisure or both or neither is intimately related to the temporal, spatial and cultural conditions in existence (p. 7).

We can see here again a link to a thread running through this book, namely the idea of time, space and culture linking together all aspects of our work and lives (see Chapter 4).

Grint cites Arendt's (1958) opposition between labour and work as a possible way forward in defining: what is work? – where labour is *bodily activity designed to ensure survival in which the results are consumed almost immediately* and work is *the activity undertaken with our hands which gives objectivity to the world.'* There are, however, problems with this definition (Grint 1991, p. 8) in that there is a difference between industrial and non-industrial societies in the outcome, e.g. immediate consumption of products is not necessary to survival in industrial societies.

Work has a 'transformatory capacity' – an activity which alters nature – whilst an occupation is a status group which locates individuals within a 'market' and stratification. Note that work and labour are interchangeable within the dictionary definition of these terms but can still have very different connotations, dependent on the context in which they are used. Grint (1991) makes the observation that:

> Work occupies a substantial portion of most people's lives and has often been taken as a symbol of personal value: work provides status, economic reward, a demonstration of religious faith and a means to realise self-potential. But work also embodies the opposite evaluations: labour can be back-breaking and mentally incapacitating; labour camps are punishment centres; work is a punishment for original sin and something we would all rather avoid (p. 1).

In focusing this chapter on nursing work (*that is the work undertaken by nurses – my focus*) we need to consider how these two definitions, as seen by Grint, have any impact on how nursing as a profession and occupation are defined. Certainly the term 'nursing' as a form of emotional labour, as defined by Pam Smith (1992) and others, is a relatively new way of considering what is involved in the work of nurses. Some of these views are discussed here but also in Chapter 8 and elsewhere.

Initially, however, we need to consider how nursing work is seen by nurses themselves as well as others who work alongside in various health care situations. It is also important to consider how the image of nursing and therefore nurses has been seen in wider society and in various cultural contexts.

Nursing work in a political and social context

The ongoing political stance on nursing and the appearance of support for its development as a profession, on one hand could be viewed as rhetoric hiding the reality, that is that the nursing hierarchy is modelling itself on the medical model of knowledge and hierarchy at the expense of its own history and its care work. On the other hand the political proposals for nursing (in the UK at least) and the still perceived challenge to medical dominance is, one could argue, one of expediency and necessity rather than one of support for development of a nursing profession, that is as there are not enough doctors to carry out doctors' ('traditional') work, they are now becoming de-skilled in certain areas as nurses become 'skilled up' and taking on what was previously considered the domain of a medical professional. Consider, for example, the role of the Advanced Practitioner – who can work in various health care situations. I am not meaning here the advanced practitioner nurse who is able to work autonomously in a nurse care role, but a trained practitioner from a number of various health care profession backgrounds especially nursing, working at a very high level of skill and knowledge, such as being capable of the highest level of medical prescribing. They can be employed in a number of contexts, such as psychiatry or in a context where they can conduct their own specialist health clinic (including advanced-level medicine prescribing) in a health care centre alongside the General Practitioner (GP). (See: https://www.hee.nhs.uk/our-work/advanced-clinical-practice for full details on this role as defined by Health Education England.)

The same kind of de-skilling or rather role merger is then taking place in nursing in relation to health care support workers, and now the nursing associate role (UK specific). This latter role after much challenge across the profession initially has now become registered by the UK Nursing and Midwifery Council (2018) and therefore governed by statute. This development became part of the ongoing debate surrounding the importance of patient safety and quality of care in the UK NHS (see earlier comments). Alongside this in 2018 the nursing professional body the Nursing and Midwifery Council (NMC) approved a major change in the nursing curricula for registration as a qualified nurse of the future where the expectations of a newly qualified nurse from 2022–2023 onwards is clearly being defined by high expectations in terms of leadership and management of care rather than necessarily being directly involved in the delivery of nursing care. These expectations are added to by the increasing number of new (to those students in the UK) clinical skills that student nurses will be expected to attain, such as chest auscultation, taking and reading ECGs, full body clinical assessment and many more (Nursing and Midwifery Council 2018, Annexe A).

The discourse as related to division of labour and roles, between medicine and nurses, has similarly taken place by authors observing the situation in the USA. The emergence of a nursing culture there has its roots in the same origin as in the UK and elsewhere, with Florence Nightingale and her work. However, it was to be much later after Florence Nightingale returned from the Crimea when nursing work in the USA became noticed, and that again was due to the outbreak of a war; in this case the American Civil War (12 April 1861–9 April 1865) (Egenes 2018; Schultz 2004). Much like the Crimean War (1853–1856) the impact of the American Civil War brought major attention to the role of the nurse and its relationship to the work of doctors.

However, in terms of nursing the sick (and defining the concept of Sick Nursing) as well as the role of the nurse, (see D'Antonio 2010 in her interpretation of the development of nursing in the USA), we can see clearly that there were similar debates on how both these roles should not only relate to each other but how nurses were being perceived as needing to be subordinate to doctors in their knowledge and practice. D'Antonio (2010) also offers an interesting narrative on a social background issue that was not, however, in the late 1880s a major part of nursing's development in Britain: that of the African American nurse, their own story of course aligned with the political context and racial tensions that was dominant at that time, and indeed much later. (See Further Reading for another edited book by D'Antonio and colleagues on nurses' work in the USA.)

If these are changes to nursing work brought about through political and professional body expectations, is there a parallel change in how the image of the nurse is seen, both inside the health care professions and by society itself? This issue of the image of nursing and nursing work has to be set against the particular society in which it exists. This is very important, which is why I have stressed that similar developments and changes discussed already in the UK are not necessarily taking place in most countries worldwide. In countries such as the USA, Australia, Canada and Sweden, for example, there are continual and ongoing nursing changes, whilst others such as India and Africa have a varied pattern of change dependent on their economy and external collaborations with countries like those already mentioned. Certainly both nursing as undertaken in the USA and in the UK has had an impact on many countries developing their nursing as both occupation and profession.

This is mainly due to the fact that nursing as care work and nursing as a profession is very much at a different level of development in many countries and not only that but how nursing as work is considered by each society itself, that is its status, is also determining its importance to the economy and to the overall health care system. Because nursing is also seen by many societies worldwide as 'women's work' this is an added challenge to its development. (See later discussion in this chapter and in Chapter 8.)

One example can be seen in the developments over time in the Russian Federation (Gerry & Sheiman 2016) where in terms of a division of labour between nurses and doctors, it has in fact been very heavily weighted towards doctors doing a majority of health care work. This has resulted in, until recently, a major proportion of the health care workforce being that of the medical profession. This has a major impact on the members of the workforce that are classed as nurses to the extent where Gerry & Sheiman (2016) state:

> It is true that, to some extent, a division of labour has now started to take place in Russia, albeit to a substantially lower degree. The predominant perception of nurses has been as an assistant to the physicians, and this has not changed much over recent decades. Therefore, the major characteristics of nurses' professional capacity have remained – the absence of theoretical knowledge, poor understanding of service delivery organization and management, and a limited area of practical skills. This is in contrast to the western trends (p. 11).

This lower status attributed to nurses in Russia's health care culture will have had a significant impact on the culture of nursing in Russia. Despite searching the grey literature and journal sources, the actual nursing curriculum for those students from Russian Federation communities remains unclear. Grant (2018), however, offers an excellent insight into the image of nursing, especially as regard to gender, over a set period of time in the Soviet Union.

Unfortunately I cannot possibly consider all the challenges impacting on nursing work in different countries worldwide in this book, but can illustrate some of the specific ones throughout key chapters. In this chapter we can consider in particular nursing work and its image in different societies and how this can impact on how the nursing role is seen generally alongside other roles such as that of the medical profession. The traditional care and cure debate is viewed alongside the division of labour in particular between doctors and nurses, as being the predominant discourse throughout nursing's history. My view is that regardless of the blurring of boundaries seen in nursing work as in the UK, and indeed between nursing and medicine, the historical image and indeed health care belief systems will continue to retain the professional boundaries between medicine and nursing, doctors and nurses. We will explore this in the next part of the chapter but also consider how nursing work can be seen through different lenses, not simply aligned against the work that doctors do, and explore some of this from different cultural contexts.

Nursing and the nurse: the images over time

I have chosen to focus initially, through an 'anthropological' lens, on the impact that aspects of Florence Nightingale's work, as related to nursing, has had on the image of nursing. We must not forget, however, that other similar figures have also had an impact on the image of nursing in different countries.

My own nursing journey for example, which began in 1967, was clearly influenced by the vocational care image, but alongside that, however, was clearly a strong view, influenced by the images emerging of women in the 1960s, that not only could I do something meaningful that I had wanted to do since a child, but that I would also receive some remuneration for 'working' as a student nurse and be able to not rely on my parents to keep me any longer.

The image was not one of receiving an education or an educated nurse but that of gaining a training which included the skills to be a 'good or excellent nurse'.

Of course, on reflection this had to have included an education through being taught theory underpinning the skills and practice we undertook on the wards. The image of being a nurse revolved around our uniforms, badges and belts, role status, correct acknowledgement of senior nurses and deference to matron and senior ward sisters! All this, of course, was enacted against the background of our role in caring for mainly sick people. This was a very rich tapestry of nursing in which we existed and one where that 'caring' image of the nurse has persisted even today, but not so the same cultural symbols associated with nurses of the past. The majority of nurses today, unless for special ceremonies, (see Chapter 2) no longer have to wear caps, belts and buckles, although there are examples from private hospitals, as opposed to public hospitals, where this happens.

In terms of how the image of the nurse has been perceived over time and therefore the work that they do, the biggest influence has been the vision of Florence Nightingale and one could argue the romanticism that still surrounds her role as 'The lady with the lamp'. Kalisch & Kalisch (1987) call it: 'The Angel of Mercy image' (p. 17), and they noted that: '*Nightingale gave to the nursing profession both an unprecedented degree of public respect and acceptance and a new and abiding symbol of excellence*' (p. 17).

Nightingale has therefore entered the folklore that surrounds nursing and also the culture of nursing as one of its major symbols. In the UK certainly her work and her life has been built into the wider education culture, through various stages of the primary education National Curriculum, but even this was threatened in 2013 by planned changes to the history curriculum, alongside removal of teaching about the other now famous British nurse – Mary Seacole. (See comments for the proposed changes by the Florence Nightingale Society: http://nightingalesociety.com/correspondence/reform-of-the-national-curriculum-in-england/ which include an interesting narrative of how these two nurses are viewed by members of the Society.)

Of course, alongside the Florence Nightingale image we had that of a Sarah Gamp-type nurse, epitomised for all time in the work of Charles Dickens (*Martin Chuzzlewit*). According to Kalisch & Kalisch (1987) Dickens played an important part in the early stages of nursing reforms and was a supporter of Florence Nightingale and her work. Here we can see the influence of the early press, through the publication of his books which included vivid portrayals of health care and social conditions of the time, as well as the essays he published (see Kryger 2012).

Regardless of how authors have portrayed their understanding of Florence Nightingale from her own writings, and early records of her work as well as others, her continued portrayal by the nursing profession internationally remains an essential part of the culture of nursing. A PhD study by Selanders (1992) of *An analysis of the utilization of power by Florence Nightingale 1856–1872*, offers a rewarding insight and analysis but also an interesting comment in her conclusion:

> The negative aspect of Nightingale's legacy is that she did not appear to empower nurses to use power in the same manner as which she did in order to effect change. As nurses struggle with power and empowerment issues, it appears that the mode of effecting change in the future must come through transformational leadership within the profession (p. 110).

As far as nursing culture is considered, however, we need to consider whether her still being seen as representing nursing is more about needing a cultural symbol that also represents not only a cultural shift about nursing itself as a vocation moving towards paid employment, but also about the shifting position of women in Victorian society.

Salender's view about Nightingale being unable to demonstrate how she acted as a direct transformational leader for nurses to be able to take control of their own futures, and therefore those coming afterward, needs to be considered alongside what she did achieve which has remained a core cultural concept: that of raising awareness and then action that regardless of how society viewed her, this same society deserved nurses that were educated and trained to give the best possible care to patients during her lifetime and, indeed, beyond.

To illustrate her influence on nursing and nursing education in other countries, I was honoured to be asked to present a paper about nursing models used in the UK at a Japanese nursing conference. Imagine my surprise to find that not only was a colleague presenting a paper on the Nightingale Model of Nursing, but that the curriculum being taught was based on this same model. (See brief reference to this model in Tokumoto et al. 2011: https://www.athensjournals.gr/health/2017-4-2-4-Tokumoto.pdf). A full-sized statue of Florence Nightingale took pride of place in the School foyer and Japanese colleagues were very interested in hearing more about her work and the possibility of visiting the UK to see her history. Takahashi (2004) offers wide-ranging examples of the influence of Florence Nightingale on the development of nursing in Japan and also how her perceived *'feminine virtues of altruism, self-sacrifice, integrity and purity were moral values for ideal women – "good wives and wise mothers" to have in the "ie" space'* (that is the family home sphere of life for a woman in Japanese culture at the time) and that as it became necessary for women to seek employment outside the home, to ensure they secured an equivalent social space to the 'ie', *'where they were not only protected, but ascribed membership and status'* (p. 56) and nursing could then be considered an acceptable employment as these *'moral qualities'* were expected to be essential qualities by the Japanese Red Cross Society and were therefore *'following Nightingale's example'* (p. 159).

Takahashi also includes a quote from **Inoue** on behalf of the Japanese Society on the Inauguration of the Florence Nightingale International Foundation (Takahashi 2004, p. 108) – who had stated the following:

> We always feel as if we too, live in London. In other words, Florence Nightingale is the idol, not only of we Japanese nurses, but also of Japanese women in general, old and young. Indeed she is deeply enshrined in the hearts of Japanese womanhood ....
>
> Her portrait is enshrined in hospitals and nursing schools. Our instance of devotion, which perhaps English people can hardly comprehend, is that of a large shrine, built in Japanese style, erected in her memory, and there she is worshipped as a goddess. Many visitors pay homage to her there. (RUHL Archives, BC/AL/335. Report of Proceedings, 1934.)

I mention this here because this idea that the notion of her status as an idol and a potential worshipped goddess, that Japanese women/nurses paid homage to, would not be comprehended the same by those in the UK, yet we know that in nursing culture in different countries, she remains an influential figure still and is enshrined in their wider culture; as in Istanbul at the Florence Nightingale Museum where her links with that country are evident, being situated as it is in the Selimiye Barracks where it is said that she stayed when she first arrived during the Crimean War. In London we also see this relationship with her nursing career through another Florence Nightingale Museum and also the famous Nightingale School of Nursing established in 1860 by Florence Nightingale herself (now of course re-established but retaining her name).

In considering the importance of Florence Nightingale herself it remains clear that her influence on the culture of nursing globally was significant and she remains an essential part of the folklore and tapestry of nursing culture. She is, one could argue, clearly still a symbol for nursing values that we should as nurses aspire to but this is now out of context with the wider social and political context in which nursing as a profession and work exists. Nevertheless she and her work retain that ultimate symbol of the nurse and what nursing is meant to stand for, and indeed possibly has perpetuated, even invisibly, the image of nursing as a vocation.

Some countries have created a way of using this for celebrating nursing through the use of 'rites of passage' ceremonies at student graduation ceremonies and the lighting of a replica of Florence Nightingale's lamp. In the UK the Florence Nightingale Foundation (https://flor ence-nightingale-foundation.org.uk/about/westminster-abbey-commemoration-service/) also uses the lamp and states that it has in fact *become an international symbol of nursing*. Her life and work are commemorated every year at Westminster Abbey with one nurse carrying the 'ceremonial' lamp supported by other nurses in a procession through the Abbey (https:// www.nursingtimes.net/westminster-abbey-welcomes-annual-celebratio n-of-nursing-founder/5084832.article). There then takes place a ceremony involving the handing over of the lamp from the nurse with the lamp to two colleagues who then pass it to the Dean of Westminster or a religious representative from the Abbey who places it on the alter. This is then followed by a short service of dedication to her work and what she represents. The inclusion of student nurses in the escort is an essential part of this annual ceremonial event, and relates to the transfer of (nursing) knowledge to future nurses.

In the traditional cultures of the world, celebration ceremonies are an essential part of retaining a sense of community and social cohesion and many such ceremonies are supported by rituals (see Chapter 5). Accessing the descriptions of the annual commemoration for Florence Nightingale it is evident that there is an exact replication of what happens at each annual service – from the time the ceremonial lamp is taken from Florence Nightingale's Chapel, with the same order or participants, until the end of the religious service (see: https://florence-nightingale-foundation.org.uk/about/ westminster-abbey-commemoration-service/).

Many similar issues are discussed in Chapters 5 and 6 and it is evident that even today there are similar ceremonies taking place not just to celebrate Florence Nightingale's contribution to nursing but also to celebrate nursing's contribution to societies worldwide.

In 2020, however, there will be international collaborations to celebrate the life of Florence Nightingale, as it will be 200 years since her birth, but most importantly it will also celebrate nurses and nursing's contribution to health care delivery and improving health globally (See: https://florencenightingale2020.wordpress.com/about-2/).

Nursing work in different cultural contexts

The book edited by Holden & Littlewood (1991) focusing on *Anthropology and Nursing* continues to give me inspiration into the possibilities of being able to explore, through an anthropological lens, the way in which nursing has been and continues to be seen in different societies worldwide. The chapter authors' historical perspectives on Ancient Greece, India ancient and modern, Japan and Uganda bring to life possibilities for engaging in my own exploration of some of these as well as new offerings.

India and Japan are two of these and having raised some of the issues with regards to her work in Japan I will endeavour to focus on India specifically, given the developing body of evidence that has emerged since Somjee (1991) published her earlier work.

There is one major theme in relation to nursing work in any country and historical context and that is the relationship or parallel development of nursing and nursing work and women's work in the home. Reverby's study (Reverby 1987, p. 1) argues that '*nursing is a form of labour shaped by the obligation to care*', that is that '*nursing as work is based on our expectation and need for someone to take up the obligation of care*' and that in order to understand its history and identity it is necessary to understand its relationship to 'womanhood'. Nursing as 'paid labour' rather than the 'domestic duty of care' is seen to be established as a result of the development of medicine and the establishment of the hospital as a place where sick people were treated (see Chapter 2).

Reverby (1987, p.1) expanded on this relationship between nursing and women's work, stating that: '*Nursing, as women's domestic labour structured by duty and custom, was very slowly supplemented by nursing as women's paid labour reshaped by marker forces and cultural changes*' (p. 1).

Alongside this shift of nursing from a culture of care to that of work was the growth in medicine's body of knowledge of disease and its treatment, requiring a need for these nurses to be trained to care for patients within this context. This now created a stronger division of labour in health in health work. Rafferty (1996, p. 25) saw this as nursing bringing the '*domestic hierarchy into the workplace* '. Carpenter (1993) had cautioned however that this division of labour between doctors and nurses was not always as it seemed, because within nursing itself there was in practice clearly a developing 'other', in terms of division of labour, as other health care workers encroached upon what had been considered nursing roles and skills and created within it '*nursing's internal division of power*' (p. 126). Of course there is more to this discourse concerning nursing, women's work and their status set against, in Oakley's terms, '*the removal of production from the home to the factory*' (Oakley 1981, p. 6), as well as its ongoing relationship with the medical profession.

The relationship between nursing, women's work and its status in a society is played out against the background of the actual position in society of women in general, and in many societies also influenced by religious and cultural beliefs.

Somjee (1991) discussed the change to the nursing profession in India and especially noted that at the time: '*People in India hold culturally conditioned stereotypes about nurses, as they do about other professions, each of which are influenced and shaped by the pace of social change within society*' (p. 37).

This was very much linked to both religion and what caste nurses belonged to, as this determined what they could undertake in terms of nursing actions in relation to sick people. Somjee (1991), however, noted that as time progressed and with the '*arrival of women from higher castes*' many of whom were married with families, and therefore '*a part of mainstream society*', talk about the '*looseness*' of nurses in relation to the intimate caring and body touching that were part of the nurses' caring role '*gradually decreased*' (p. 39). (Some of these issues related to pollution and handling of the human body and its excretions are found in Chapter 8.)

Hadley et al. (2007) conducted a study to determine why Bangladeshi nurses avoid 'nursing' as direct patient care in hospitals in Bangladesh. In particular they *'identified conflict between the inherited British Model of nursing and Bangladeshi societal norms'*, and in particular in the areas of night duty, contact with strangers and involvement in 'dirty work' (p. 1166). Those interviewed said that the public associated their activities 'with commercial sex work'. Interestingly they found that they used 'nursing surrogates' to carry out some of their work because of 'social conflicts faced by nurses' but also most importantly that the culture in hospitals added to these conflicts, preventing any possibility of a positive change in caring for the sick by nurses. Hadley & Roques (2007) had also conducted another study focusing on observational activities in medical and surgical wards in Bangladesh hospitals. This had established key issues regarding their lack of direct contribution to care in certain key areas of nursing practice, but the study concluded that a decision was needed as to the *'appropriateness of a Western Model of nursing in Bangladesh society'* (p. 1164).

Nair (2012) in her study focusing on gender, status and migration of nurses in India, in particular the migration of nurses from Kerala, found that some of the perceptions of Indian nurses were still influencing nursing work, despite major changes in nursing education and the work environment. The stigma for anyone working with bodily fluids and sick bodies remains linked to pollution and purity issues but also related to their position in society as being women undertaking care work. She points out, however, that it is not just in this kind of cultural context in India that these prejudices exist, that in fact *'the stigmatization of nursing is global'* (p. 192). Interestingly a major doctorate study of Johnson's (2011) still found that despite the change taking place in the nursing education system and enhanced working conditions:

> while nurses are connected by shared concerns around a stigmatized social identity and a desire for collective social mobility, tensions within the profession were found to contribute to a 'fractured professional identity'. This was marked by intergenerational differences, divisive accounts of nursing in public and private institutional settings and competing visions for the future of Indian Nursing (p. 200).

However, the most surprising issue for me was her assessment of the value still placed on the beliefs and values of Florence Nightingale, whose legacy she saw as still exerting a *'considerable influence over nursing culture in India'* (p. 200). This she said was a: *'striking feature of the research data on professionalising strategies'*. Johnson (2011) was also very clear on how this was evidenced and that: *'Within the discourse of nursing leaders, Florence Nightingale was promoted as the "ideal nurse" that all nurses should aspire to and whose life served as a point of reference in the development of nursing'* (p. 197).

Johnson initially did not understand how this *'symbol of Indian nursing's British past could exert such a strong influence upon nursing culture in India'* (p. 198). She concluded, however, that in transmitting, for example, the values espoused by Florence Nightingale, in particular to student nurses, that in fact she *'provides a strong sense of a "professional consciousness" for nurses in India and is used as a cultural anchor to bring the profession together'* (p. 198).

Here we see yet another example of Florence Nightingale as an 'icon' for the nursing profession. Her impact on nursing as care work is clearly international, and when we consider what in any culture and its language is representative of this image by others, then clearly Florence Nightingale has come to represent nursing's cultural image. Whether this is no longer a realistic vision of a nurse or indeed nursing in most societies is irrelevant in a cultural sense, one could argue that we all need to have a sense of our past in order to move forwards to a future in a culture that has learnt to manage change. I find the phrase used by Johnson above about Florence Nightingale in India, that she is '*used as a cultural anchor to bring the profession together*', very insightful and this is possibly why the ceremonies such as the annual celebration at Westminster Abbey (see page 71) are important, not just for those who can attend or take part in the main ceremony. It is a kind of reaffirmation of our cultural inheritance and an acknowledgement of how we come to be as nurses in society and brings people together for that reason. As in many cultures where ceremonies are part of the pattern of daily life, this particular ceremony, according to my discussion in Chapter 5, is clearly a ritual given its fixed content, the people who take part, the religious affirmation and the symbolic lamp.

However, we need to be very mindful that we (nurses and nursing) are also seen to be a profession, that is one where our work is remunerated and that has a specific status afforded to us by the title *nurse*. This requires us to be registered by a professional body such as the Nursing and Midwifery Council in the UK, and informs people that in using that title of *nurse (registered as such)* we have to uphold certain expectations laid down in law.

This state registration for nurses (1910) was the result of a successful campaign fought by Mrs Ethel Bedford Fenwick, against the views of doctors and others such as hospital administrators at the time (Rafferty 1996) who perceived a threat posed by women (at the time fighting for their rights to vote) and importantly by Florence Nightingale herself.

The issues involved in their ongoing pursuit of what was necessary for nurses and therefore nursing itself are unfortunately beyond the scope of this chapter. However, one can only imagine where nursing would be today in a political and social sense if both these women had worked together for the benefit of nurses. It is, however, clear to see from the literature where the issue of training (as per Florence Nightingale and learning on 'the job' and 'how to do the job', as well as documenting their experiences) and education as for a respected (professional) occupation (as per Mrs Bedford Fenwick and learning by doing similar activities to those espoused by Florence Nightingale but with the major difference being the written passing of exams and theory and then being acknowledged through registration) could appear to be two separate and opposing views. Rafferty (1996) offers an invaluable insight into the many debates encountered around training and education of nurses by these two women, and others, at various periods of time since then. Most importantly, however, these insights are set against the political and social context of the time. Both women had an impact on the future of nursing, yet only the one has been retained as the symbol of nursing that focuses on the vocational expectations and moral standing expected of a 'good' nurse. Her very image of the Lady with the Lamp caring for patients in Scutari is a reminder that a nurse's role is caring for the sick and those unable to care for themselves. The appearance of other now considered 'famous' nurses such as Mary Seacole, for example, are to be seen for different reasons for their contribution to the development of nursing (see Further Reading).

The reality today, however, is that whilst it remains symbolic of what nursing has stood for, nursing work today requires much more than this one image. We have abandoned most of the 'trappings' associated with the symbol of a nurse as seen by nurses in Florence Nightingale's era and beyond (see Chapter 5) yet it is difficult to see what or who can replace such an individual as a cultural representation or symbol of what nursing means today. We have seen the issues still facing nurses in countries such as India, where in fact Florence Nightingale has been seen to be a symbol for change for women who wish to become nurses (Johnson 2011).

Conclusion

I began this chapter by trying to establish what was the core of nurses' work as it relates to a nursing culture. It is evident, however, that despite a common understanding of what nursing involves in relation to caring for the sick in society, in fact the most fundamental impact on nursing culture is how the wider society in which it exists impacts on the world of those who are called nurses. It is evident across global cultures that nursing has a specific role to play in societies, and where there is a common understanding when mentioning the word nurse, of what that means as an image. The fact that societies worldwide also identify with Florence Nightingale as the ultimate historical image of what a nurse stands for remains intact. She has become a cultural symbol for nurses worldwide and clearly all these various ceremonies and celebrations of her life and work, one could argue, maintain our inherent vocational beliefs about the role that nurses have in relation to others but also that nurses can achieve, with the right skills and knowledge, a major cultural shift in how nursing as a profession is seen in any society. Nursing work in some cultures remains a challenging occupation but possibly those nurses now need to build their future not just around cultural symbols but through an enhanced understanding of what is important for nurses and those they care for in their own society.

References

Arendt H (1958) *The Human Condition.* University of Chicago Press, Chicago. Cited in K Grint (2005) *The Sociology of Work: Introduction*, Polity Press, Cambridge.

Carpenter M. (1993) The subordination of nurses in health care: Towards a social divisions approach. In E Riska & K Wegar, *Gender, Work and Medicine: Women and the Medical Division of Labour*, 95–130, London, Sage.

Coast E (2000) *Maasai Demography*, Unpublished PhD study, University College London, London.

D'Antonio P (2010) *American Nursing: A History of Knowledge, Authority and the Meaning of Work*, John Hopkins University Press, Baltimore.

Egenes K (2018) History of Nursing. In G Roux & J A Halstead, *Issues and Trends in Nursing: Practice, Policy and Leadership*, 2nd Edition, Chapter 1, 3–30. Jones & Bartlett Learning, Burlington.

Gerry C J & SheimanI (2016) *The Health Workforce of the Russian Federation in the Context of the International Trends*, National Research University Higher School of Economics, Research Paper No. WP BRP 01/PSP/2016, (https://wp.hse.ru/data/2016/12/02/1113380342/01PSP2016.pdf).

Grant S (2018) *Nurses in the Soviet Union: Explorations of Gender in State and Society.* In M Ilic (ed) *The Palgrave Handbook of Women and Gender in Twentieth-Century Russia and the Soviet Union*, Chapter 17, 249–265, Palgrave Macmillan, London.

Grint K (2005) *The Sociology of Work: Introduction*, Polity Press, Cambridge.

Hadley M B, BlumL S, Mujaddid S, Parveen S, Nuremowla S, Haque M E & Ullah M (2007) Why Bangladeshi nurses avoid 'nursing': Social and structural factors on hospital wards in Bangladesh, *Social Science and Medicine*, 64, 1166–1177.

Hadley M B & Roques A (2007) Nursing in Bangladesh: Rhetoric and Reality, *Social Science & Medicine*, 64, 1153–1165.

Holden P & Littlewood J (1991) *Anthropology and Nursing*, Routledge, London.

Johnson S E (2011) *A 'Suitable Role': Professional Identity and Nursing in India*, Unpublished PhD study, London School of Hygiene and Tropical Medicine, London. (https://researchonline.lshtm.ac.uk/834552/1/550402.pdf, accessed 6 May 2019).

Kalisch P A & Kalisch B J (1987) *The Changing Image of the Nurse*, Addison Wesley, Menlo Park, California.

Kryger M (2012) Charles Dickens: Impact on Medicine and Society, *Journal of Clinical Sleep Medicine*, 8 (3), 333–338.

Nair S (2012) *Moving with the Times: Gender, Status and Migration of Nurses in India*, Routledge, London.

Nursing and Midwifery Council (2018) *Regulation of Nursing Associates*, NMC, London. (See the NMC Council Decision at: https://www.nmc.org.uk/globalassets/sitedocuments/councilpapersanddocuments/council-2018/council-papers-sep-2018—na-papers.pdf, accessed 12 May 2019.)

Oakley A (1981) *Subject Women: A Powerful Analysis of Women's Experience in Society Today*, Fontana Press, London.

Rafferty A M (1996) *The Politics of Nursing Knowledge*, Routledge, London.

Reverby S M (1987) *Ordered to Care: The Dilemma of American Nursing 1859–1945*, Cambridge University Press, Cambridge.

Schultz J E (2004) *Women at the Front: Hospital Workers in Civil War America*, University of North Carolina Press, Chapel Hill.

Seccombe I, Smith G, Buchan J & Ball J (1997) *Enrolled Nurses: A Study for the UKCC*, Institute of Employment Studies, Brighton.

Selanders L C (1992) *An Analysis of the Utilization of Power by Florence Nightingale 1856–1872*, Unpublished PhD study, Western Michigan University, Michigan.

Smith P (1992) *The Emotional Labour of Nursing*, Palgrave Macmillan, Basingstoke.

Somjee G (1991) Social change in the nursing profession in India. In P Holden & J Littlewood (1991) *Anthropology and Nursing*, 31–55, Routledge, London.

Takahashi A (2004) *The Development of the Japanese Nursing Profession: Adopting and Adapting Western Influences*, Routledge, London.

Tokumoto H, Goto K & Arai M (2011) Reflecting on clinical training instruction: Improving new instructors' capabilities, *Athens Journal of Health*, 4(2), 155–168.

Further reading

1   Allen D (2007) What do you do at work? Professional building and doing nursing, *International Nursing Review*, 54, 41–48.

2   D'Antonio P, Baer E, Rinker S D & Lynaugh J E (eds) (2007) *Nurses' Work: Issues across Time and Place*, Springer, New York.

3   Davies C (1976) Experience and dependency and control in work: The case of nurses, *Journal of Advanced Nursing*, 1, 273–282.

4   Ehenreich B A & English D (2010) *Witches, Midwives and Nurses*, 2nd Edition, The Feminist Press, New York.

5   Hawkins S (2010) *Nursing and Women's Labour in the Nineteenth Century: The Quest for Independence*, Routledge, London.

6   Leeson J & Gray J (1978) *Women and Medicine*, Tavistock Publications, London.

7   Mackay L (1989) *Nursing a Problem*, Open University Press, Milton Keynes.

8   McDonald L (2018) *Florence Nightingale, Nursing and Health Care Today*, Springer, New York.

9   Melia M (1984) Student nurses' construction of occupational socialization, *Sociology of Health and Illness*, 6(2), 132–151.

10 Reverby S (1987) A Caring Dilemma: Womanhood and Nursing in Historical Perspective, *Nursing Research*, 36(1), 5–11.

11 Smith P (2012) *The Emotional Labour of Nursing Revisited: Can Nurses Still Care?*, 2nd Edition, Palgrave Macmillan, Basingstoke.

12 Towell D (1975) *Understanding Psychiatric Nursing: A Sociological Study of Modern Psychiatric Nursing Practice*, RCN, London.

8

DIRT, POLLUTION AND THE BODY

Meaning for nursing practice

Karen Holland

Introduction

In many of the other chapters in this book you will already have seen reference to these words 'dirt' and 'pollution' as they refer to nursing and nurses' work. You may, if you are a nurse reading this, also have had the experience of friends or family members who may ask the question on 'how can you do that job, with such dirty things to do, like emptying bedpans and wiping patients' bodies?'. The question of how both female and male students 'manage the bodies' of patients of their opposite gender is often a real concern for students who embark on nursing as a career, but especially those that may have no previous experience in a health worker role. Both roles are associated with the body in terms of what nurses have to physically do in terms of managing body 'products', but also as seen in many cultures, how men and women are viewed in terms of their traditional role expectations when also being a nurse. As seen in Chapter 7, the view of nursing as women's work which is seen as 'dirty work' has a major impact on the status of nursing across different societies.

In addition there are strict 'taboos' associated with being a woman in most societies, in relation to their normal bodily functions, such as menstruation and pregnancy, which in addition can also be influenced by the religious beliefs of their communities. We must not forget, however, that nursing is no longer defined by its female gender past, but that men are now more visible in their role as student nurses, as undertaking the same work is a pre-requisite to becoming a qualified nurse. Whether that work is sustained in their post-registration employment remains to be seen, and we will certainly be exploring some of those issues in relation to what Simpson & Simpson (2018) refer to *as 'the intimate and messy bodily care work of nursing'* (p. 5).

In this chapter I will explore some of the evidence that will raise an awareness for the reader of how the main issues of dirt and pollution, especially in relation to the body, impact the way nursing care (as care work) is both seen and managed by nurses, but also the views of the societies in which they live and work.

It is clear from my research for this book that these two concepts have a major impact on how nurses are both viewed in society as well as how this is then translated into their work.

Yet I was surprised to see that these views and explanations have come not, in the main, from the nursing community but rather from sociologists and anthropologists who have made a study of these issues of dirt and pollution as related to a wide range of types of care work generally. Nursing and its historical development, of course, has been a rich environment for such studies.

Before exploring some of these issues it is very important that we all begin with an initial understanding of how these concepts of dirt and pollution are evidenced in the anthropological literature, as well as how the body is also contextualised in relation to them. We will begin with the body because we can then position the key issues related to dirt and pollution as related to nursing work, and indeed the position of nursing and nurses, in various societies as a direct result of their relationship.

The body and anthropology

Where to begin exploring this topic was not an easy decision, until I recalled where I had undertaken a similar experience in studying for the MSc in Medical Social Anthropology. One of our course tutors set us a task of exploring a personal body experience using concepts from anthropology. This we agreed was a seemingly daunting task but one which my colleagues and I of course made every attempt to complete and to put into practice what we had learnt. I chose, on reflection afterwards, something possibly too personal and complex in relation to what had been my 'bodily' experiences of being a woman, but which had to be placed in an anthropological context.

Like then I begin with a very brief description of what is a body, using Synnott's (1993, p. 1) definition as a starting point:

> Breasts, thighs, lips, eyes, heart, belly, navel, hair, penis, nipples, arms, brain, guts and balls. Body parts: but also much more. We have imposed layers of ideas, images, meanings and associations on these biological systems which together operate and maintain the physical body. Our bodies and body parts are loaded with cultural symbolism, public and private, positive and negative, political and economic, moral and often controversial ... the body is not just skin and bones, an assemblage of parts, a medical marvel ... the body is also, and primarily the self. We are all embodied.

We can already see from this definition that the body is more than our body parts, yet together they are inextricably linked into how we not only view ourselves but also how others see us and often how we use the body to express ourselves, how we see others' bodies and in some situations how our bodies are either managed or controlled. For this chapter, however, we are focused on how a view of the body and indeed body 'products' are an essential part of our understanding of the work of the nurse, but also how this impacts on how others perceive that work in various societies (see also Chapter 7).

Synnott (1993) in his important work on *The Body Social*, includes an important chapter on The Body and Senses (p. 228) where he explores a range of sociological and anthropological theories on how the body and bodies are seen and how they give us insight into how societies both use their bodies as an integral part of their cultural beliefs and symbolism, but also how these theories can help us to understand that a person's body is more than the physical and external. The nurse in her work of course has to 'manage' the physical body as it were in undertaking a number of care practices, but most importantly, in addition the work of the nurse also involves the caring (nursing) for the whole person which one could relate to Synnott's own view of the body as the self. That is more than the physical external body self but we will see in a later theorist view, what many nurses are taught about, which is the mind of the person, how they feel about things, how they see their illnesses, how they communicate their beliefs about their health and of course how they see their physical body and what is going wrong with it when they are sick. All of these are essential to a nurse being able to carry out their work as nurses in the best way for the patient and their needs. This is of course a very simplistic explanation but for now it is helpful in beginning a discussion about mainly anthropological theories concerning the body. There is clearly, from my reading, often a blurring between sociological and anthropological theories in relation to the body, but I will endeavour to focus on the latter and offer recommendations for further reading at the end.

To ensure that we can at least gain an insight into the basic concepts of how the body is seen anthropologically, we can look at some of the main theories, as does Synnott (1993), beginning with the view of the body as discussed by the anthropologist Mary Douglas (1970).

Mary Douglas and the body

Her work on *Purity and Danger* (Douglas 1966) focused on rituals, and a relationship to hygiene, dirt and pollution in various societies. Mary Douglas continued her interest in the body in various cultures as well as how it can be used in various symbolic ways, and her work entitled *Natural Symbols* (Douglas 1970) included her developing theories about how meanings can be attributed to the body and based on her extensive anthropological experience.

The idea of the 'body' as being two concepts in one is viewed by Mary Douglas in a very different way to that I described earlier. She introduces us to an anthropological view of the body with her theory of the '*two bodies*', namely the self and society, the body social and the body physical. She refers to these also as the 'self and society', one related to the body as related to an external social sense and the other the actual physical body. She states that often the 'social body', and by inference our existence as a human being in our own society, creates pressure on how the 'physical body' is perceived or indeed can actually exist in our society. In terms of what we need to focus on as nurses, it is not only how the physical self/body is viewed but most importantly how anything that relates to this body is actually managed.

Again we can begin to see an emergence of how societal views and pressure impacted, for example, on the work of Florence Nightingale and her nurses and how they were seen by the wider social community in Victorian times, especially in Britain; their 'angels of mercy' image and vocational calling conflicting with perceptions of what they were tasked with in relation to caring for the wounded and the sick during the Crimean War.

What they saw and what they had to undertake within the actual context of their work was, one could argue, normalised in that localised context in Scutari and other nearby hospitals for example (see the account of *Eastern Hospitals and English Nurses* by an unnamed author – A Lady Volunteer 1856), and only became seen as not normal in fact when the reality and nature of their work became known outside this context, and then their work symbolised something entirely different. This was not only reflected in their work in handling the body and body products but also in the fact that as women they undertook tasks that involved the management of the patients as men in the wider social context, that is the 'social body'. The Victorian restrictions on how men and women ought to conduct themselves in relation to each other in social situations had a major impact on how they were to conduct themselves within the home as both wives and mothers. The account by the author known as A Lady Volunteer highlighted this in her account of nurses working in hospitals on the Bosphorus: when many of the paid nurses eventually returned home, many of them were refused employment because they had been engaged in military hospitals and there was much confusion on the nature of the work some had carried out. Also many of the nurses had illness and sickness themselves which was an added issue. A particular statement about the unreal social and cultural context that nurses, doctors and other carers lived in together, brings to mind how their situation might be viewed by others: '*The life in the East was eminently calculated to bring out the whole bent of a person's character, for it was destitute of all help and restraint which the ordinary rules of English society afford*' (p. 346).

There are many books exploring the work of Nightingale and her nurses in relation to how their work in nursing was seen, especially the self sacrifice for the good of others and their position in society (Hallam 2000; Hawkins 2010) but none specifically focusing on it with an anthropological lens. Gamarnikow (1991), however, explored how the Nightingale system of nursing created hierarchies within the profession but also how nursing began to create a more autonomous role as separate from their medical colleagues' influence (see p. 112). Her focus related to the societal view of nursing as women's work and the occupational division of labour with doctors, which then impacted on the kind of work nurses could undertake, especially in relation to cleaning. Garmanikow (1991) explains how this changed as: '*Nursing reform redefined nursing as healing. Thus, cleaning became the nurse's contribution to hygiene and patient welfare*' (p. 115).

So in relation to Mary Douglas's '*two bodies*' view, you can begin to consider how it can help us understand in particular the (physical body) work of nurses in their unique social situations and what kind of issues impact on societal expectations and indeed perceived images of nursing work.

Although I have used a very brief insight into how that could possibly be viewed in the era of Florence Nightingale's nursing, we can still see similar patterns remaining in today's nursing culture across many societies (see Chapter 7, for example, on nursing in India).

Another view of the body that is relevant to consider here is that of medical anthropologists Nancy Scheper-Hughes and Margaret Lock. Their paper entitled *The Mindful Body: A Prolegomenon to Future Work in Medical Anthropology* (Scheper-Hughes & Lock 1987) embarks on a major review of the anthropology of the body but they make it clear that '*despite its title this article does not pretend to offer a comprehensive review*' but, as the title suggests, a starting point for future discourse on the body (p. 6). They focus the extensive paper around their view of what they term 'The Three Bodies' in that:

> At the first and perhaps most self-evidence level is **the individual body**, understood in the phenomenological sense of the lived experience of the body-self.
> At the second level of analysis is **the social body**, referring to the representational use of the body as a natural symbol with which to think about nature, society and culture, as Mary Douglas (1970) suggested. At the third level of analysis is **the body politic,**

referring to the regulation, surveillance, and control of bodies (individual and collective) in reproduction and sexuality, in work and in leisure, in sickness and other forms of deviance and human difference (p. 7–8: **my focus in bold**).

They also state importantly that:

> Conceptions of the body are central not only to substantive work in medical anthropology, but also to the philosophical underpinnings of the entire discipline of anthropology, where Western assumptions about the mind and body, the individual and society, affects both theoretical viewpoints and research paradigms. These same conceptions also influence ways on which health care is planned and delivered in Western societies (p. 6).

In an attempt to explore briefly their view of these three bodies I will use some of the work I wrote as a personal experience essay using anthropological concepts, where in fact this paper was a major starting point in unpacking my own '*body experience*' over time. I refer to one particular issue (**menstruation**) as it relates to one of my next sections on pollution, and is an issue that both nurses and midwives can refer to.

In terms of the individual body, mine had been originally defined by its sex and became subsequently a mirror of my cultural existence in terms of my gender. Caplan (1987) informed us that a widely used distinction is made between sex in the physiological sense and gender which is a cultural construct. So for the first 11 years of my life I lived in this ascribed body of a 'female'. However, at age 11 a life-changing experience took place with the onset of menstruation, a symbol if you like that my body was making a transition to maturity. However, this bodily function had an outcome every month – with the 'red blood flow' of a menstruating body. Not only was it a shock that this was to happen every month but that I had to take care of this bodily outpouring myself. Of course I was not the only one this was happening to and also not just in my country but to girls and women worldwide. I recall that at these monthly times, I excluded myself from swimming with my brother and sister in the sea and got a letter from my mother to excuse me from physical activities in school. The fear or anyone knowing that I was in fact 'bleeding' became initially a serious concern. I did not, however, have to be separated from anyone as a necessity.

In some societies and cultures menstruation becomes a situation that requires seclusion rituals for the menstruating girl/woman. La Fontaine (1985) describes what happens in the Wogeo tribe regarding this, whereby:

> While menstruation cleanses women, the blood itself is polluting and a woman must not come into contact with people or property while she is in this condition, nor touch the food of her husband lest he die. She is secluded in her hut; must keep warm and observe food taboos; uses a hole in the wall or in the raised floor, not the usual door, when going out to urinate or defecate; wears a special skirt which proclaims her polluted status and must use special instruments to eat or drink with (p. 127–128).

Of course there is much more involved in the overall ritual related to menstruation than this brief insight, and indeed in this Wogeo society described by La Fontaine, there is a parallel experience that men undergo that also creates a blood-related ritual.

At menstruation the third body described by Scheper-Hughes and Lock becomes very visible, the body politic. It is a transition which could end in possible pregnancy and childbirth. I found an interesting paper by Goodale (1980) with regards to how the Kaulong consider menstruation and childbirth, in that they are considered to be periodic illnesses, similar in fact to the medicalisation of these 'normal' female functions in Western societies. From their view of a 'healthy body', i.e. intact mind, self and the body, one can identify that any loss from the body could be considered unhealthy. The woman is therefore particularly dangerous and a source of pollution, but rituals ensure that the 'polluting female' is made known to the men. A woman is not allowed anywhere near drinking water and supplies and '*she may not touch anything with which a man may come into contact*' (p. 129). The Kaulong believe that '*female pollution is dangerous only to males*' (p. 130). Goodale offers more insight into this culture and their beliefs and, despite its age, it is a paper very worthy of reading in terms of considering comparisons in how the body politic is played out in other cultures when it relates to women and their reproductive functions. Unfortunately I am unable to pursue more discussion on this issue of menstruation as polluting. (See Holland 2017, Chapter 6: Women and healthcare in multicultural society, p. 95–113.)

Blood itself has a kind of symbolic association for many people, outside of menstruation taboos, certainly in nursing and health care, as with life and death situations where we see patients needing large volumes of blood to be able to survive. It is symbolic then of saving a life. However, blood can also be considered the reverse and dangerous to others as we have seen in the past with the HIV virus (seen in Wiley et al.'s (1990) study of nurses' concerns of being infected), and Hepatitis C which can impact the health of the patient and, if care is not taken with blood products by nurses, such as when removing blood from the patient during care and treatment, could also cause potential harm to the nurse.

Despite research and education worldwide there are still fears about the dangerous effect of blood. A study by Wada et al. (2016) took place in Japan and their conclusion was that although there was still some reluctance to care for some infected patients with HIV/Hepatitis C, there was an overall '*lack of confidence in taking precautions against these diseases*' (p. 6).

However, currently in the UK there is taking place a major inquiry into how infected blood came to be used for people in seemingly 'normal situations' where blood was required, e.g. for patients with haemophilia requiring blood transfusions. The stories of lives ruined due to stigma associated with having to declare that they were infected are being related and reported, as well stories of many who have experienced death or dying relatives from this infected blood being made public. Fear of what blood can do other than save lives is yet again back on the public agenda. (See the Hepatitis C Trust for ongoing updates on this inquiry as well as new reports on the impact of the virus by patients and nurses: http://hepctrust.org.uk/blog/mar-2017/hepatitis-c-patients-and-nurses-highlight-impact-virus-new-reports).

Blood in these situations has been translated into being harmful (or indeed polluting) to a person with, in many cases, serious outcomes. The life-and-death scenario is vividly told in peoples' stories of their experiences or those of others in televised interviews or narratives for the social media and press.

Bharj (2007), for example, wrote an interesting paper using in particular the work of Mary Douglas to explore how midwives could themselves be considered to be polluting (defiling) South Asian women within the childbirth experience and we shall be returning to this and other similar issues in the section on pollution.

So what do we mean by pollution or polluting? In much of the literature there is also a strong link to dirt and their meaning and relationship to each other.

Dirt and pollution: some anthropological observations

Douglas (1966) states that *'our idea of dirt is compounded by two things, care for hygiene and respect for conventions. The rules of hygiene changes of course, with changes in our state of knowledge'* (p. 8). Simpson et al. (2012) explain Douglas's view that in fact *'dirt and pollution is "matter out of place", that is arising when there are violations of cultural norms or of the social order'* (p. 3). Douglas (1966, p. 44) offers examples of this view of dirt as *'matter out of place'*, and that *'it implies two conditions: a set of ordered relations and a contravention of that order. Dirt then, is never a unique isolated event. Where there is dirt there is system.'*

She then offers contextual examples of how we may see this notion of order in relation to dirt and what happens to that view when the order of things is upset. I think that these will resonate with many readers:

> Shoes are not dirty in themselves, but it is dirty to place them on the dining table; food is not dirty in itself, but it is dirty to leave cooking utensils in the bedroom, or food besbattered on clothing; similarly, bathroom equipment in the drawing room; clothes lying on chairs; outdoor things indoors; upstairs things downstairs; under-clothing appearing where over-clothing should be and so on. In short, our pollution behaviour is the reaction which condemns any objective or idea likely to confuse or contradict cherished classifications. (pp. 44–45)

I can certainly hear myself saying to my grandchildren comments such as 'if your shoes are dirty leave them in the porch, don't bring them into the house', or 'please put that empty yoghurt pot in the bin when you have finished and then wash your hands'.

These types of sayings have been learnt over time and are part of the normal pattern of daily life, as it were, in certain households, unlike some cultures where the issue of what can be taken into a house or left outside is an essential part of that society's cultural beliefs about health and illness. An example of this is Japanese culture. Ohnuki-Tierney (1984) offers an excellent insight into the way in which the concept of dirt and therefore what is clean is managed in Japanese society. She begins by saying that: *'Daily hygiene practices are based on one of the most fundamental concepts in any culture: what is clean and what is dirty'* (p. 21).

These daily hygiene practices are focused around taking shoes off and washing hands, and in some families Japanese children are also taught *'to gargle when they come into the house from the outside'* (p. 21). The main focus to their hygiene activities is to keep dirt 'outside' the home and *'to keep oneself clean and healthy "inside" in one's own living quarters, one must get rid of this dirt thorough cleansing'* (p. 22).

Hendry & Martinez (1991) offer an additional insight into this inside and outside aspect of daily life in Japan, and like Ohnuki-Tierney, who states that a *'hospital is one of the dirtiest places, where the dirt of others is concentrated'* (p. 26), they tell us that *'hospitals are by definition full of germs … and also peopled with outsiders'* (p. 58).

Simpson et al. (2012) stress, however, that *'cleanliness and dirt are therefore not just material matters but can have social and moral significance, triggering with respect to dirt a desire to avoid or remove it and stigmatising those who are involved in it'* (p. 3).

However, they also offer explanation that not all dirt is seen as 'equally polluting', offering the example by Dick (2005), who points out cases where certain bodily fluids are seen as contaminating 'dirt', that '*avoidance rules mean that occupations which deal with polluting, physical dirt are carried out by members of lower classes, who are separated spatially and socially from other groups*' (such as 'untouchables of the Hindu class system), whereas those from higher-status occupations dealing with similar dirt (such as doctors) have avoidance rules about what they can and cannot be in close contact with.

This issue of dirt and its polluting effect on the physical body is also translated into the context of the hospital whereas, as Littlewood (1991) pointed out, the sick in society are contained, and therefore everything associated with them is also contained so that others are not contaminated. She refers to some of what nurses are expected to do, such as nursing work related to clearing up '*faeces, urine and vomit*' as '*sick dirt*' and '*so highly polluting that they would not be removed by domestics*' (p. 178). She also states that '*nurses become intimately involved and identified with the containment of personal pollution*' (p. 178).

Wolf's (1988) book published from her doctorate work, called *Nurses' Work: The Sacred and the Profane*, focused on her findings that there existed four nursing rituals (see Chapter 5) linked to '*nurses' work as both sacred and profane*' (p. x) and her description of a procedure that many nurses take for granted, namely the bath, presents it as an example of purification of the body. It is evident from an earlier paper that Wolf (1993) had undertaken an in-depth analysis of how the bath was not only considered by her a nursing ritual but that the practice was very much linked to hygiene and dirt as expressed by Douglas.

The body, dirt and pollution in nursing work

We now need to consider how the issues already explored can be seen in the context of nursing work and especially as it impacts on the role of the nurse. I have found already in my reading that to do justice in terms of words and space in this chapter, I will have to keep focused on key issues. This section, although interlinked conceptually, will focus on these key areas: Nursing as body work, Nursing as Dirty Work and Managing dirt, pollution and the body in nursing.

Nursing as body work

I found two examples that can be used to define what is meant by this view of nursing as 'body work'. Wolf (2014) stated that:

> Nursing work is historically and culturally viewed as 'bodywork'. Despite efforts to professionalise nursing practice through education, practice changes and collective organisational effort, in the public's eye the work of nurses continues to be inextricably bound to the physical care of patients' bodies (p. 147).

Twigg et al. (2011) support this link to patients' bodies by focusing on what this could look like for different health care professionals in the field of health and social care, but as seen from their broad definition this view expands beyond the notion of managing the physical care of patients' bodies, whereby:

Body work is work that focuses directly on the bodies of others: assessing, diagnosing, handling, treating, manipulating and monitoring bodies, that these become the object of the worker's labour (p. 171).

I do not intend to focus on these wider issues here, as both papers expand their content to include sociological concepts in relation to body work, some along the lines of Scheper-Hughes & Lock's (1987) third body – the body politic. Both papers, however, are essential reading in relation to the reader's understanding of their impact on how nurses manage the 'physical' body (Douglas 1970) and the individual and social bodies explored by Scheper-Hughes & Lock (1987).

Picco et al. (2010) raised an issue about human uniqueness with regards to corporeal identity. Using the work of Merleau-Ponty they noted that: '*Each human being possesses a body distinct from those of another human being: the body renders a person unique and allows the individual to perceive his/her world and so establish continuous relationships with it*' (Merleau-Ponty 1994, p. 39).

For the nurse caring for a patient in a variety of health care situations, the importance of recognising the uniqueness of that person is an essential part of their professional practice.

In reading this paper by Picco et al. (2010) I recalled a book I used in my teaching, about the concept of body image, by Bob Price (1990), which offered an invaluable way of explaining to students how they could view issues of body image they may encounter in practice and how they could then support the patient. I managed to locate the book and was drawn again to his ideas regarding the body. He explained that his definition of body image contained three components, whereby '*human beings throughout life attempt to sustain balance*' between the three as follows:

> … body image is the way in which we perceive and feel about our body (**body reality**), how it responds to our command (**body presentation**) and includes an internal standard by which we are judged (**body ideal**) (p. 4).

Obviously he proceeds to expand on each of these but when we consider how nurses need to respond to aspects of body work in their practice, alongside their understanding of how to care for the physical body and the way it works in both health and illness, then it is essential to recognise that the person or individual self's view of their body in the first place is an essential part of nursing the whole person. I found also that when exploring further these three aspects of body image, I could also relate them to the 'social body' and the 'body politic'. For example, *body reality* '*refers to our body as it really is*', for example short or tall, fat or thin (Price 1990, p. 5); *body ideal* '*is measured constantly against an ideal of what we think a body should look like and how it should act*' (p. 6) and he explains that within this concept is also how we consider body space and boundaries. One example he offers here is in terms of how patients on mechanical ventilators lose their ability to define '*their usual body boundaries*' and that '*the machine tubing can come to be seen as part of the body – the machine an extension of personal body space*' (p. 7). Body ideal also relates to how our body functions, and some people will actually become distressed when, for example, the reality of their physical body is altered in some way so that their body ideal is no longer a possibility. Imagine, for example, a young person who has to have bowel surgery requiring the permanent positioning of an external colostomy (where the bowel is actually now on the body surface), where the products of digestion now appear in a bag outside the body. Not only has their body reality changed but also their view of a body ideal. In terms of how this will be possibly viewed by others in society, this is clearly a situation of '*matter out of place*' and where the '*two bodies*' could be said to collide (Douglas 1970).

Body presentation at its simplest level is '*how we present our body appearance to the social world*' and we are able to control this '*within certain limits and to reflect actively in how body presentation was received by others*' (Price 1990, p. 11). Imagine how a person may feel about a changed body appearance, when they are required to put on a hospital gown during an intimate examination or to go to the operating theatre for surgery. Their normal (private) body decisions become secondary to the more public reality that their body is now exposed to, and on view to, others.

However, from personal experience of going to the operating theatre, the focus is more on what will happen there rather than being concerned too much about what one looks like in what is stated to be a 'clean' gown. Of course, entering the operating theatre lying on a trolley, one is immediately struck by the fact that this is meant to be a 'sterile' and non-polluting environment, from the way in which everyone is colour coded to their occupied spaces, and again from experience there are those who are on the periphery who are called 'the dirty nurse', who undertake to remove, for example, 'surgical waste products' considered unsafe to the patient and the physical environment, and ensure that the area and the people around the patient are kept as sterile and dirt free as possible.

Katz's (1981) paper offers a detailed anthropological insight into this environment, in her exploration of '*ritual in the operating room*', where she explains the '*separation of realms of cleanliness (sterility, asepsis) from realms of pollution (non sterility, sepsis, contamination)*' (p. 349). There are clear distinctions between one and the other.

Creating ritual is also highlighted by Philpin (2007) in her explanation of how nurses '*manage danger, uncertainty and ambiguity in ITU through avoiding or protecting themselves from pollution*' (p. 55). They wear protective clothing, masks, gloves and in some cases goggles in order to prevent infection to the patient, but also to themselves, as in the operating theatre many patients not only need to be kept from harm but they themselves are also a potential polluting risk to the nurse.

Philpin (2007, p. 57) offers an example of this, and also how nurses cannot always separate out their own 'selves' as it were when faced with a potentially polluting experience, through this field note excerpt:

> As I helped 'Elizabeth' to turn her patient, the patient suddenly vomited copious amounts of foul-smelling, thick faecal fluid. Her lips, face and pillow were covered in this liquid. 'Elizabeth' was so overcome with nausea; she was very pale, sweaty and gagging uncontrollably, had to leave the bedside.

Philpin (2007) explains this scenario: '*This was an extreme and visually shocking example of matter out of place – faecal fluid on the face, lips and pillow – that was impossible not to also experience on an olfactory level*' (p. 57).

Lawler (1991), in her now seminal research work published as *Behind the screens: Nursing Somology and the Problem of the Body*, brings a whole new insight into nursing as body work and body care; in particular how student nurses have to learn to overcome situations as did

Elizabeth in Philpin's study; also, how to manage the 'body' of their patients, for example, when undertaking their first bed bath. One of her informants (Lawler 1991) highlights this through talking about this first experience:

> We are taught the proper way to carry out a bed bath, but not how to deal with the breaking of the social taboos when we wash a patient's body …. As a young female you work with a patient (who might well be male) behind drawn curtains and are expected to strip and wash his whole body (p. 119).

In this section I have offered an insight only into issues of nursing as work related to the body and body care. There is, of course, much more detail and depth that we could explore and I have offered you further reading to supplement further interest and evidence.

However, although I have alluded to issues of pollution, dirt and cleanliness there is a need to consider these in more detail as a balance to the issue of how nurses manage and care for the patient as both the 'physical body' and their 'embodied self'. It is important to note as well that to illustrate much of our understanding of both I have in the main focused on the person who is experiencing illness and has a disease (Kleinman et al. 1978), where the issue of the care of the body is more acute. However, some nurses have also to manage not just physical illness but also the care of the patient who has an acknowledged mental (health) illness, sometimes with a physical illness/disease but often on its own. Here, body care and body work take on an entirely different experience.

Nursing as dirty work

We have already explored aspects of body work by nurses set against theories of dirt and pollution but it is essential that we now focus on how nursing has been seen as 'dirty work', despite its variable status in different societies. What does dirty work actually mean?

Both Simpson & Simpson (2018) and Simpson et al. (2012) focus on the impact that Everett Hughes has had on defining this in an organisation sense, as well of course as Mary Douglas anthropologically. According to Ashforth & Kreiner (1999), Everett Hughes (1951) *'invoked the term "dirty work" to refer to tasks and occupations that are likely to be perceived as disgusting or degrading'* (p. 413). They offer a typology based on Hughes' later work (Hughes 1958) to support their exploration of 'meaning and social significance of dirty work' (p. 414), in particular as it relates to three forms of taint: physical, social and moral taint. By considering Ashforth and Kreiner's explanation of these three we can begin to see how in fact nursing is impacted by at least two of the three, and in some countries possibly three. They note that:

> *physical taint* occurs where an occupation is either directly associated with garbage, death, effluent and so on … *social taint* occurs where an occupation involves regular contact with people or groups that are themselves regarded as stigmatised e.g. prison guard, HIV/AIDS worker, social worker, psychiatric ward attendant … *moral taint* occurs where an occupation is generally regarded as somewhat sinful or of dubious virtue, e.g. exotic dancer, pawnbroker or others such as police interrogator (p. 415).

They do add two specific provisos to this typology – namely that:

dirtiness is a social construction: it is not inherent in the work itself or the workers but is imputed by people, based on necessarily subjective standards of cleanliness and purity. Secondly – the common denominator among tainted jobs is not so much their specific attributes but the visceral repugnance of people to them (p. 415).

Recall the beginning of this chapter when I considered being asked: how can you do that job (i.e. nursing)? These issues of taint and dirtiness can clearly be seen in how nursing is viewed as a job in itself in a society, and also how those who undertake the work are actually seen by others in that same society. In particular, is there a difference in how men in nursing work are seen to that of women? Simpson (2009) offers an interesting perspective of the male nurse in relation to their perceived body, as initially how men, because of their physiognomy and size, manage difficult and potentially violent situations and are able to offer their physical strength to assist a patient that a smaller female nurse may not be able to manage. However, this view of a male nurse could have implications in terms of how intimate female care should be managed (p. 108) but highlights how one nurse managed this:

> Dealing with or working with females on surgical wards, gynae wards, my managers went through great problems to work out whether I needed a chaperon or not to do a procedure on a female patient. I thought how stupid, I'm a nurse. It doesn't matter whether you're male or female, you've got the skills and the knowledge to do a procedure (p. 108).

Simpson et al. (2012) explore this aspect of the male nurse's work through a study undertaken in Australia. One point made which we have seen in other studies is the issue of male nurses entering more managerial-type posts and thereby removing themselves from the direct contact with the 'body work' inherent in the traditional role of the nurse. They also offer further insight into those aspects of taint mentioned earlier with examples, and I offer one here, regarding physical taint:

> *Dead bodies – it's not nice dealing with all that. At first I found it quite disturbing – repellent really. But at the end of the day, you just have to get on with it. Perhaps it's a male thing – you quite literally have to roll up your sleeves and do it* (General nurse).

How then is what Douglas and others talk about with regards to dirt, dirtiness, cleanliness and pollution, especially in relation to the body of a person, in all its aspects as discussed, managed in nursing and related work?

We know already that the nurse has to manage and care for the physical body, but they also have to manage those products that are part of normal health, such as urine and faecal matter, when a person is ill.

It is important that we consider some understanding of what we mean here by being ill and refer to Young's (1982) reference to the work of Arthur Kleinman et al. (1978) who categorised how one could consider disease, illness and the later sickness, in the following way:

> DISEASE refers to abnormalities in the structure and/or function of organs and organ systems; pathological states whether or not they are culturally recognized; the arena of the biomedical model. ILLNESS refers to a person's perceptions and experiences of

certain socially disvalued states including, but not limited to, disease. SICKNESS is a blanket term to label events involving disease and/or illness. According to Kleinman, medical anthropologists need to remember that their domain is sickness, even though their special contribution will be mainly with regards to illness (Young 1982, p. 264).

Jervis (2001) undertook an ethnographic study in a US inner city nursing home, and in particular focused her paper on the work of nursing assistants, which she stated was in '*many ways, prototypical "dirty work" and that as primary caregivers to the sick, the "crazy" and the dead in nursing homes, nursing assistants are constantly threatened with becoming symbolically polluted*' (p. 84). She determined that the main threat to caregivers' '*sense of self and status on the job*' was incontinence care. We can also see this possibility of being symbolically polluted in relation to the role of the nurse in other situations, not just in a similar nursing home context observed by Jervis.

Wolf (1986), for example, makes it clear that '*nurses' dirty work involves direct contact with bodily products, including secretions and excretions, and with products of infection*' (p. 29) but also notes that '*few outside of nursing or within nursing, explicitly label nurses as dirty workers*'. However, we also know that based on what has been discussed in this chapter, nursing work has retained this perception that nurses deal with the unpleasant aspects of people's lives when they are sick. This involves intimate care and managing body fluids that normally a person would be managing themselves in their own home.

It is unclear from my research for this book how care of the patient who remains sick, but does not require hospital care and is cared for by district nurses, for example, is viewed, as their sickness is contained not in a hospital as Littlewood states but actually within their own home. Twigg (1999) offers an interesting view of how the balance of public and private as regards bathing and washing is disturbed when disability happens, and that the normal 'dedicated spaces within the home' may no longer be available to manage these normally private aspects of body care.

Nurses attending them to offer care and treatment such as wound dressings still have to deal with infection control and to ensure that neither the patient nor others are 'polluted' by dirt or 'germs' which could cause harm.

One practice that happens in both hospital and the home is making sure the patient is bathed or bathes themselves. Some parts of the body are considered dirtier than others, with Wolf (1986) pointing out that '*the face is cleaner than the hands and feet and the genitals and perianal areas dirtier than the abdomen and back*' (p. 31).

When it comes to washing a patient who may be incontinent of urine and faeces, for example, I recall being taught as a student nurse that one must always wash from clean areas to dirty body areas, and in fact often washing the genital and perianal areas would be undertaken by the patient themselves if they could manage this, in order to save them embarrassment – especially if an older man or a woman – given that I would have been only 18 years old at the time!

An important statement by Wolf (p. 31), however, related to what Florence Nightingale began regarding hygiene and the importance of cleanliness: '*Absolute cleanliness has been demanded of the nurse for over a century. The dirty work of nursing is juxtaposed with the clean work of nursing.*'

Wolf also stresses this view in relation to personal cleanliness and Florence Nightingale and ensuring that the patient is safe from harm, but also that nursing work also overlaps with religious areas (sacred work) and moral and ethical values which remain an essential part of nursing and their professional codes of conduct worldwide.

Conclusion

This chapter has focused on the way in which nurses manage dirt, pollution and the body in nursing. Keeping to an anthropological lens, however, was not without its challenges, as much of the research and theories on the body in health care work generally as well as nursing were focused on the sociological. The content of this chapter is an essential part of our understanding of nursing not just in terms of how these concepts appear to influence nursing work, but also the status of nursing in various societies worldwide.

We like to think that nursing in fact, in terms of the work that nurses do, has come a long way in terms of what actually happens in practice but in reality the core of nursing in relation to the sick in society remains. There are challenges in that much of nursing is changing, for example less direct nursing in terms of body care and work being undertaken by qualified nurses, as well as the role of the patient in their own care.

Given the nature of societies and indeed sickness, illness and disease, the nature of some nursing work as clean and some as dirty will continue to be an area that requires further understanding. An anthropological lens has offered us a brief insight into the relationship between one and the other, alongside how they both relate not only to the body of the person but also the body of the nurse.

References

A Lady Volunteer (1856) *Eastern Hospitals and English Nurses*, 3rd Edition, Hurst & Blackett Publishers, London. Reprinted in the BiblioLife Reproduction Series.

Ashforth B E & Kreiner G E (1999) "How can you do it?": Dirty work and the challenge of constructing a positive identity, *The Academy of Management Review*, 24(3), 413–434.

Bharj K (2007) Pollution: Midwives defiling South Asian women, In M Kirkham (ed), *Exploring the Dirty Side of Women's Health*, Chapter 4, 60–71, Routledge, London.

Caplan P (ed) (1987) *The Cultural Construction of Sexuality*, Routledge, London.

Dick P (2005) Dirty work designations: How police officers account for their coercive force, *Human Relations*, 58(11), 1363–1390.

Douglas M (1966) *Purity and Danger: An Analysis of Concept of Pollution and Taboo*, Routledge, London. Routledge Classic Edition published in 2002.

Douglas M (1996) *Natural Symbols: Exploration in Cosmology*, 2nd Edition, Routledge, London.

Gamarnikow E (1991) Nurse or woman: Gender and professionalism in reformed nursing, 1860–1923. In P Holden & J Littlewood, *Anthropology and Nursing*, 110–129, Routledge, London.

Goodale J (1980) Gender, sexuality and marriage: A Kaulong Model of Nature and Culture. In C P MacCormack & M Strathern, *Nature, Culture and Gender*, Chapter 6, 119–142, Cambridge University Press, Cambridge.

Hallam J (2000) *Nursing the Image: Media, Culture and Professional Identity*, Routledge, London.

Hawkins S (2010) *Nursing and Women's Labour in the Nineteenth Century: The Quest for Independence*, Routledge, London.

Hendry J & Martinez L (1991) Nursing in Japan. In P Holden & J Littlewood, *Anthropology and Nursing*, Chapter 4, 56–66, Routledge, London.

Holland K (2017) *Cultural Awareness in Nursing and Health Care. An Introductory Text*, 3rd Edition, Routledge, London.

Hughes E C (1951) Studying the Nurse's Work, *The American Journal of Nursing*, 51(5), 294–295.

Hughes E C (1958) *Men and their Work*, Free Press of Glencoe, Illinois.

Jervis L L (2001) Pollution of incontinence and the dirty work of caregiving in a US nursing home, *Medical Anthropology Quarterly*, 15(1), 84–99.

Katz P (1981) Ritual in the operating room, *Ethnology*, 20(4), 335–350.

Kleinman A, Einsberg L & Good B (1978) Culture, illness, and care: Clinical lessons from anthropologic and cross-cultural research, *Annals of Internal Medicine*, 88, 251–258.

La Fontaine J S (1985) *Initiation: Ritual Drama and Secret Knowledge Across the World*, Penguin Books, Harmondsworth.

Lawler J (1991) *Behind the screens: Nursing, Somology and the Problem of the Body*, Churchill Livingstone, Edinburgh.

Littlewood J (1991) Care and ambiguity: Towards a concept of nursing. In P Holden & J Littlewood (1991) *Anthropology and Nursing*, Chapter 10, 170–189, Routledge, London.

Merleau-Ponty M (1994) *Phenomenology of perception*, Routledge, London. Italian translation 2003, *Fenomenologia della percezione*, Bompiani, Milano.

Ohnuki-Tierney E (1984) *Illness and culture in Contemporary Japan: An Anthropological View*, Cambridge University Press, Cambridge.

Philpin S M (2007) Managing ambiguity and danger in an intensive therapy unit: Ritual practices and sequestration, *Nursing Inquiry*, 14(1), 51–59.

Picco E, Santorio R & Garrino L (2010) Dealing with the patient's body in nursing: Nurses' ambiguous experience in clinical practice, *Nursing Inquiry*, 17(1), 39–46.

Price B (1990) *Body Image: Nursing Concepts and Care*, Prentice Hall International (UK), Hemel Hempstead.

Scheper-Hughes N & Lock M (1987) The Mindful Body: A Prolegomenon to Future Work in Medical Anthropology, *Medical Anthropology Quarterly*, 1(1), 6–41.

Simpson R (2009) *Men in Caring Occupations: Doing Gender Differently*, Palgrave Macmillan, Basingstoke.

Simpson R, Slutskaya N, Lewis P & Hopfl H (2012) Introducing dirty work, concepts and identities. In R Simpson, N Slutskaya, P Lewis & H Hopfl, *Dirty Work, Concepts and Identities*, Chapter 1, 1–18, Palgrave Macmillan, Basingstoke.

Simpson R & Simpson A (2018) "Embodying" dirty work: A review of the literature, *Sociology Compass*, 12, e12581.

Synnott A (1993) *The Body Social: Symbolism, Self and Society*, Routledge, London.

Twigg J (1999) The spatial ordering of care: Public and private in bathing support at home, *Sociology of Health and Illness*, 21(4), 381–400.

Twigg J, Wolkowitz, Cohen R L & Nettleton S (2011) Conceptualising body work in health and social care, *Sociology of Health & Illness*, 33(2), 171–188.

Wada K, Smith D R & Ishimaru T (2016) Reluctance to care for patients with HIV or hepatitis B/C in Japan, *BMC Pregnancy and Childbirth*, 1–6, 16(31) (https://bmcpregnancychildbirth.biomedcentral.com/articles/10.1186/s12884-016-0822-2#Abs1).

Wiley K, Heath L, Acklin M, Earl A & Barnard B (1990) Care of HIV-infected patients: Nurses' concerns, opinions, and precautions, *Applied Nursing Research*, 3(1), 27–33.

Wolf K A (2014) Critical perspectives on nursing as bodywork, *Advances in Nursing Science*, 37(2), 147–160.

Wolf Z R (1986) Nurses' work: The sacred and the profane, *Holistic Nursing Practice*, 1(1), 29–35.

Wolf Z R (1988) *Nurses' Work: The Sacred and the Profane*, University of Pennsylvania, Pennsylvania.

Wolf Z R (1993) The bath: A nursing ritual, *Journal of Holistic Nursing*, 11(2), 135–148.

Young A (1982) The anthropologies of illness and sickness, *Annual Review of Anthropology*, 11, 257–285.

Further Reading

1 Anderson B (2000) *Doing the Dirty Work? The Global Politics of Domestic Labour*, Zed Books, London.

2 Bashford A (2000) *Purity and Pollution: Gender, Embodiment and Victorian Medicine*, Macmillan Press, Basingstoke.

3   Ben-Ari E, Moeran B & Valentine J (eds) (1991) *Unwrapping Japan: Society and Culture in Anthropological Perspective*, University of Hawaii Press, Honolulu.
4   Bolton S C (2005) Women's work, dirty work: The gynaecology nurse as 'other', *Gender, Work and Organisation*, 12(2), 169–186.
5   Hahn R A (1983) Rethinking "illness" and " Disease ", Contribution to Asian Studies, Vol XVIII, p135–157
6   Hallam E, Hockey J & Howarth G (1999) *Beyond the Body: Death and Social Identity*, Routledge, London.
7   Hendry J (2013) *Understanding Japanese Society*, 4th Edition, Routledge, London.
8   Kirkham M (ed) (2007) *Exploring the Dirty Side of Women's Health*, Routledge, London.
9   Kleinman A (1989) *The Illness Narratives: Suffering, Healing, and the Human Condition*, Reprint Edition, Basic Books.
10 Lawler J (1997) *The Body in Nursing*, Churchill Livingstone, Edinburgh.
11 Lawton J (1998) Contemporary hospice care: The sequestration of the unbounded body and 'dirty dying', *Sociology of Health & Illness*, 20(2), 121–143.
12 Lupton D (2012) *Medicine as Culture: Illness, Disease and the Body*, 3rd Edition, Sage, London.
13 Rudge T & Holmes D (eds) (2010) *Abjectly Boundless: Boundaries, Bodies and Health Work*, Ashgate Publishing, Farnham.
14 Twigg J (2000) Carework as a form of bodywork, *Ageing and Society*, 20, 389–411.
15 Van Dongen E & Elema R (2001) The art of touching: The culture of 'body work' in nursing, *Anthropology and Medicine*, 8(2/3), 149–162.

9

WITHDRAWAL OF TREATMENT IN THE CRITICAL CARE UNIT

Insights into a trajectory of dying and death

Jenni Templeman

Introduction

This chapter will collate studies focusing on the anthropological insights and the sociology of dying and death in the critical care unit. It will explore issues relevant to end-of-life care, withdrawal of treatment, ethical decision making, and ritual from an anthropological perspective within the critical care milieu. A scenario of withdrawal of treatment in the critical care unit will highlight the sociological and anthropological literature and offer insights into the meanings and understanding of the conceptual aspects of uncertain death, awareness of dying, liminality, spatiality and the symbolism of bedside curtains. The critically ill patient 'becomes' the domain of the nurse, and defines the limits of a nurse's activity, emotions and lived world while in the ICU.

Symbolically, a critically ill patient who is about to undergo withdrawal of treatment may be perceived to inhabit a liminal time frame, a 'betwixt and between' state, a state of social limbo. During the orchestration of withdrawing treatment, the dying patient, the nurse and family are perceived to be on a shared liminal journey. In this parallel liminal state, the patient, family and the nurse accompany each other in a parallel 'betwixt and between' state, between life and death. Death is perceived as a disturbance of the social order, a laceration of the social body, and a gap in social and family networks. In a curative, rescue culture of critical caring, death may appear to be viewed as an enemy and sometimes perceived as a disease rather than a way of life.

The patient's trajectory of dying and death unfold behind closed curtains around the patient's specific bed space. When closed, the curtains serve as a protective, restricted 'traffic light' entry and an exit point and symbolically shield the feelings and emotions of the people behind them. The trajectory of dying and death will be explored in relation to nurses' behaviour and their role in the dying experience of the patient and supporting family following the decision to withdraw treatment.

In order for the reader to be able to see this dying and death trajectory in context, I will draw on various aspects of my doctoral study, exploring through an ethnographic lens what happens following a withdrawal of treatment decision in the critical care unit. (See Further

Reading for access to the full study.) Firstly and most importantly is describing and discussing aspects of the context in which this study took place.

The critical care scene: a unique cultural space

The critical care unit (CCU) is a sequestered area separate from the rest of the hospital, and its ambience suggests it is a place where a concealed community of practitioners delivers advanced healthcare to a specific patient profile. These medical and nursing practitioners are a hidden 'tribe' inhabiting a world of their own, armed with an arsenal of expert knowledge, experience, advanced skills and innovative therapies in the quest to stabilise and rescue critically ill patients from the 'brink of death'. The patient profile is characterised by critical illness and a multitude of disease entities which require advanced biotechnological support and specialised care. Seymour (2001) suggests that, globally, death in the CCU is characteristic of a complex and contradictory milieu. The critical care environment represents the modern preoccupation with the mastery of disease entities, the eradication of untimely death, the prolongation of life and attempts to enhance dignified end-of-life care (Seymour 2001).

On entering the CCU, one soon discovers a constant hive of activity; a purposeful flow of movement, staff talking and working, ventilators breathing, invasive flashing lights, buzzing and beeping syringe drivers, gurgling suction machines, renal haemofilters whooshing, phones ringing and different priority alarms triggering when patient parameters change beyond normal pre-set limits.

This constant motion of people moving to and fro throughout the day and night symbolically appears to reflect the waves of life, generating the eternal heartbeat of the CCU milieu, pulsating with each patient's heartbeat – a continuous ebb and flow of life and sadly often death. Turnbill et al. (2005) described the intensive care unit as a clinical space which mirrors the notion of an intense world of hope, recovery and cure, as well as disappointment and loss. Surrounding each patient's bed space is an electronic, kinetic 'state of the art' bed and an adequate bed space with a collage of highly technological computerised monitoring systems, mechanical ventilators, renal filtration machines, and a vast array of infusion pumps and syringe drivers. The beds are occupied by patients lying sedated, motionless and silent, attached to various machines with lines, tubes and monitoring devices penetrating all areas of their bodies. Consultant anaesthetists are responsible for the ultimate care of all the patients in the CCU flanked by experienced critical care nurses and a multi-disciplinary team of physiotherapists, dieticians, pharmacists and radiographers.

Decisions pertinent to each patient's treatment plan and therapeutic options are discussed and assessed in a methodical and pragmatic fashion, based on the available evidence and in the best interests of the patient on the daily CCU morning round. In the UK, every critically ill patient is afforded the opportunity to receive biotechnological life-sustaining therapies during their critical illness, unless admission to CCU is contra-indicated. At the beginning of each patient's intensive care journey family members offer and share information relevant to the patient's individual characteristics and life prior to their critical illness. This information serves to metaphorically clothe the patient's personality as they lie silently in the bed attached to various life-supportive devices and therapies. During this journey the nurses are immersed in the intensive caring of a critically ill patient whilst also supporting a family, which often induces in the nurse feelings and a sense of belonging directed towards the family.

Nurses bridge the gap between the patient and their family during withdrawal of treatment and help the family to reconnect with the dying patient. Creating an ambience of comfort and compassion during the patient's dying trajectory will directly impact on the memories that family will have for the rest of their lives.

Although the CCU represents a place where critically ill patients are treated with life-sustaining therapies to potentially reverse their illness, when a patient no longer responds to maximum life-sustaining treatment, then the decision-making issue of withdrawing treatment arises.

Decision to withdraw treatment

When maximum medical supportive therapies are no longer effective, the decision to withdraw treatment is discussed based on the ethical principle of futility. Guidelines for withdrawal of treatment in the UK are clearly set out in a document compiled by the Intensive Care Society (ICS) which suggests medical treatment should be founded on compassion and in the best interests of the patient, with effective communication, collaboration and agreement between multi-disciplinary colleagues, patients (where possible) and families (Intensive Care Society 2009). Prior to commencing withdrawal of treatment, the significance of the patient's poor prognostic factors must be explained and discussed with the family, allowing them time to come to terms with their impending loss. The final decision and responsibility remains vested in the consultant in charge of the CCU and the current law within the UK allows a competent and experienced physician to make this decision to withdraw life-sustaining treatment (Intensive Care Society 2009). The responsibility of managing the withdrawal of treatment resides with the nurse at the bedside (Coombs et al. 2010). British nurses are more autonomous in their clinical practice as compared to some of their European counterparts (Latour et al. 2009).

It is imperative that the views of the patient (if known) and the family are considered during the decision-making process to avoid conflict at this sensitive and emotive time. Withdrawing treatment from critically ill patients may be viewed as a form of euthanasia in different countries and cultures. However, the Intensive Care Society (2009) stipulates that euthanasia is illegal in the UK and plays no part in the withdrawal of life-sustaining treatment from critically ill patients.

Patients with chronic illnesses experience numerous exacerbations, only to be rescued from the brink of death by sophisticated technological interventions in the ICU (Miller et al. 2001). This unpredictable nature of chronic illness disguises the dying trajectory, creating what Callahan (1995) refers to as the vanishing line between life and death, where death is no longer experienced as a natural outcome, but rather as an inadequately treated disease, a failure of modern medicine. This viewpoint is often apparent among medical and nursing staff when the decision to withdraw treatment is taken.

Drawing the curtains and creating a space for dying

Throughout withdrawal of treatment, nurses perceive the patient's bed area as a protected space where the closed curtains shelter the patient, nurse and family from the rest of the critical care unit, other patients, personnel and clinical activities. The patient's trajectory of dying and death unfolds behind closed curtains around the patient's specific bed space and when closed, the curtains serve as a protective, restricted entry and exit point.

Vouzavali et al. (2011) and Cypress (2011) suggest a reciprocal and emotional relationship between the nurse, patient and family is fostered around the bed space throughout the patient's critical care journey. From a caring perspective, the patient's bed space appears to represent an outer, spatial dimension and an inner existential dimension (Olausson et al. 2014). Permission needs to be obtained first when entering a patient's bed space behind closed curtains, almost as an unspoken rule.

Curtains are closed around the patient's bed space on different occasions, such as caring for or assessing a patient, implementing therapies, conducting procedures, during multi-disciplinary assessment, and after the decision is made to withdraw treatment.

Bryan (2007) suggests that death is hidden in the acute hospital setting by closed curtains, and according to Costello (2006) the phenomenon of death in hospital is cloaked in secrecy. The closed curtains almost symbolically shield the feelings and emotions of the people behind them. The concept of closed curtains thus serve to protect everyone else in the critical care unit from having to witness the patient's dying and death (see also Chapter 5).

Awareness of dying

The patient is usually unaware of their own dying due to their critical illness, together with an induced sedative and analgesic state which is administered to optimise comfort and alleviate pain during the patient's critical illness. A dichotomy may exist between the action to allow death to unfold 'naturally', which attributes death to the patient's body, and to almost hastening death through withdrawal of treatment, which attributes death to the nursing practice of withdrawing treatment. Once life-sustaining therapies have been withdrawn, the patient's haemodynamic status deteriorates rapidly and in this poor output state the dying trajectory soon becomes established. The process of withdrawing treatment is a strategic practice where advanced life-sustaining technology is slowly withdrawn to almost mimic the 'natural' decline of death in accordance with prescriptive norms concerning the proper course of natural dying. Seale (1998) elicits death is not always a popular discussion theme in our death-denying culture and society, yet it remains a pivotal aspect of our social life.

Medical technology therefore becomes constitutive of the natural to the extent that it frames and determines dying and death by slowly unfolding, and in this way offering a space for the family to start grieving and the presentation of a less dramatic death (Mohammed & Peter 2009). By removing the life-sustaining technology from the patient during treatment withdrawal, the patient's dying may be perceived symbolically as a process of being given permission to die, which is socially more acceptable and therefore shifts the responsibility of death away from nurses who operationalise the actual withdrawal. Within this rescue culture of clinical practice, death appears to be viewed as an enemy and sometimes perceived as a disease rather than a way of life.

Nurses view the death of a patient as less traumatic if the patient dies a good death which is perceived as uncomplicated (Pattison 2011). Usually throughout the withdrawal of treatment process, the dying patient is still attached to the ventilator with all invasive lines left *in situ*, especially the sedative and analgesic infusion lines, because this is how the family have become accustomed to seeing the patient.

Seymour (2001) describes how dying and death in the ICU are not merely technical matters which involve issues of cost and statistical significance when patient recovery is the least likely outcome; withdrawing treatment necessitates moral and ethical consideration. Nurses and doctors often view the challenge to sustain life as rewarding and feel that when curative care changes to end-of-life care, this reward no longer exists. These critical care practitioners feel that they have somehow 'failed to rescue and save the patient'. This perspective is echoed by Seale who views death as: *'no more than an extreme example of disease'* (Seale 1998, p. 77).

During withdrawal of treatment, nurses face a dichotomy situation where they intellectually rationalise the decision to forgo treatment of the critically ill patient as a palliative measure to prevent further burden from unwarranted treatment (Rocker et al. 2010).

The CCU reflects a social life world comprising critically ill patients, advanced technology and expert practitioners where ritual and evidence-based practice co-exist within clinical practice. Perhaps the most effective rituals arise from the depth of our human experience (Chambers & Curtis 2001), and in the modern climate of advanced technological nursing, nurses often struggle to find ways to give form and meaning to dying and death within the critical care milieu. Holland (1993) suggests ritual is used as a vehicle for social change and may be viewed as protection from anxiety, maintaining social order through reinforcing cultural and social structure, and understanding its survival through change. Rituals performed by nurses control the clinical environment where the nurses often find comfort in their familiarity with the advanced technology, and the use of this technology enhances the family's confidence that everything is being done for the patient. This technology provides nurses with a tool for seeking meaning out of critical illness and death. Ritual, therefore, serves as a social defence system protecting nurses against the anxiety that is caused by human suffering (Suominen et al. 1997; Chambers & Curtis 2001). (See also Chapter 5.)

The 'good death'

A tension sometimes exists between maintaining life and relieving suffering associated with inappropriate prolongation of life due to the nature of critical care clinical practice (McMillen 2007). Since the advent of the intensive care specialty in the early 1960s, the need to address complex issues arising in clinical practice has been prevalent especially regarding the contemporary issue of withdrawal of life-sustaining treatment from critically ill patients. The 'uncertain/unknown' dying trajectory identified by Glaser & Strauss (1965) as the least likely route to death in the 1960s not only posed a problem for doctors and nurses caring for critically ill patients following withdrawal of treatment (Seymour 2001). It also influenced wider societal dilemmas regarding end-of-life decision making and providing a 'good' death (Seymour 2001). Although medical and nursing practitioners in the CCU often view death as an enemy from a curative, rescue focus of care, Kirchhoff et al. (2006) postulate that most Americans fear how they will die, rather than death itself. The modern medical view perceives individual patients as no more than carriers of multiple disease entities, according to Seale (1998).

In *Limits to Medicine*, Illich (1976, p. 106) states: *'[I]ntensive care is but a medical priesthood struggling against death.'*

Despite Illich (1976) suggesting that one cannot die a good death with technology, Pattison (2004) argued that humanistic care, despite medical technology, can be brought about by human agency in critical care and expert nursing care that reconciles technology and dying. I believe that the nurses' use of the 'therapeutic self' affords a fusion between technological and bodily dying in that it is a powerful influence in promoting a good death in the intensive care environment. The authors Seymour (2001) and Pattison (2004) contend that a critically ill patient can die a good death whilst in the CCU if the patient's treatment involves dignity and holistic care. However, creating a conducive environment for dying to occur in a busy CCU is always going to be a challenging reality. Within the critical care milieu, death has almost been tamed by an array of medical, surgical, technological and pharmaceutical interventions which serve to 'buy time' for patients with life-threatening illnesses. Advanced technology, skilled personnel, defibrillators, ventilators, cardiac monitoring equipment, and drugs to save lives and avert death surround each patient's bed space in the CCU (Hockey et al. 2010). Death is viewed as a disturbance of the social order, a laceration of the social body, and a gap in social and family networks.

Liminality

From a cultural perspective, Miller et al. (2001) suggest that death is viewed through the lens of biomedical knowledge due to medical advances changing how, when, and where people die. In the past, death was a routine part of a person's life: the presence of death and its associated rituals went unchanged for centuries, as friends, family and the community gathered to share the experience and create meaningful respect in the recognition of a dying person. However, medical science appears to have replaced religion and nature in providing a conceptual framework for understanding dying and death where it is not viewed as a natural life event, but rather a disease to be treated and conquered (Miller et al. 2001).

Philpin (2007) highlighted the coexistence of ritual and symbolism within the technical and research-based elements of critical care nursing. An uncertainty surrounds the boundary between life and death in the ICU, a situation which is further complicated by the fact that life, in this instance, necessitates life-sustaining therapies using various types of invasive technology and advanced haemodynamic monitoring. Philpin's analysis of ambiguous boundaries in the CCU relates to the anthropological concept of liminality described in the original work by Van Gennep in 1909 and states that in his theory of rites of passage (Van Gennep 2004), the liminal state ('ambivalence') refers to a stage between separation from normal life and preceding re-incorporation back into the community. The critically ill patient who is about to undergo withdrawal of treatment may be perceived to inhabit this liminal state, a 'betwixt and between' state, between life (albeit sustained by technology) and death (which ensues following the withdrawal of life-sustaining therapies). During the orchestration of withdrawing treatment, the dying patient, the nurse and family could be perceived to be in a state of liminality as described by Van Gennep (1909), and on a shared liminal journey. During this withdrawal process, the patient, nurse and family are therefore in a 'betwixt and between' state, between life and death, a tripartite liminal journey towards death. The nurse who institutes the withdrawal of treatment is aware of the patient's impending dying trajectory, whereas the patient is usually unaware of their own death due to the analgesic and sedative infusions administered and their haemodynamically labile status.

Van Gennep (1909) identified three rites of passage: the rites of separation, transition and incorporation. During withdrawal of treatment the rite of separation has occurred and the patient is in this transitional betwixt and between state, a state of 'social limbo' which

Turner (1969) describes as neither in one state nor another – a state between life sustained by technology and an impending death. The nurse's liminal state during the management of withdrawing treatment is also 'betwixt and between' life and death, as the nurse withdraws life-sustaining therapies in an attempt to 'mimic' the natural process of dying. Nurses are positioned on the threshold between life and death as they manipulate sedative and analgesic infusions during this state of social limbo. Death is omnipresent; the time, however, is unknown.

Holland (1993) highlights the importance of the liminal phase in Turner's (1969) analysis of ritual as a reinforcement of the social order and as a source of social change in the death of the patient. The nurse accompanies the patient and supports the family during this dramaturgical dying trajectory from the onset of withdrawal of treatment until death. The patient's care is concluded after death by performing the post-mortem care. This is the nurse's final contribution to the care of the patient.

Spatiality and temporality

Nurses are present at the patient's bedside 24/7, embracing the patient with intelligent observation, holistic patient assessment, and planning and implementation of the various treatment regimens. This sense of closeness and ownership denotes the nurses' focus of time and temporality, as well as the presence in a special 'space' or spatiality shared with the critically ill patient. The therapeutic use of self, temporality and spatiality are salient aspects within the nurse's remit. The patient is not perceived as a medical case, but as an individual with a life filled with meaning. Nurses become involved with their patients emotionally and almost a part of their world. This emotional involvement makes it possible for the nurse to respond to the family in a sensitive and meaningful way (Seymour 2001).

Space is multi-dimensional and provides both housing and refuge (Vouzavali et al. 2011). In clinical practice, time spent with a critically ill patient is awash with forceful experience, implicit encounters and strong feelings impenetrable to others. Symbolically, an intimate bond exists between the nurse and patient as a unity where the nurse and patient occupy the same space in a certain time. Spatiality and temporality within the context of hospital life is also evident in the patient's critical illness journey, critical care encounter and during the dying trajectory following the decision to withdraw treatment. As the nurse manages the withdrawal of treatment from the patient, the temporal and spatial aspect of the dying trajectory unfolds around the confines of the patient's bed space, where death is a certainty but the time to death remains uncertain (see also Chapter 4).

Hallam & Hockey (2001) explored the notion that death is a disturbance of the social order, a laceration of the social body, and a gap in social and family networks. Aries concludes by positing the image of medicalised death as the icon of the 'bad' death where the 'death of the patient in hospital, covered with tubes, is becoming a popular image of macabre rhetoric' (Aries 1974, p. 614). Nurses attempt to alleviate the anxiety experienced by the patient's family regarding this strange environment by explaining and educating them regarding these multiple invasive technologies and therapies from the outset when the patient is admitted to the CCU. This is an attempt to keep the family informed of the day-to-day management of the patient and to socialise them into this strange and frightening environment. The longer the patient's stay in the CCU, the more informative and familiar the critical care milieu becomes for the family. The patient is unaware of the surrounding environment due to their critical illness, sedative and analgesic status. This induces a state of unconsciousness or social limbo where the patient is also rendered aphonic due to the insertion of an artificial airway. Technological life support creates an interlude during which people strive to harmonise their understandings, expectations and plans for the patient. Family members often need time to overcome denial that the patient is dying, disbelief that treatment options no longer exist, or the restoration of healthy family dynamics.

Social death

Walter believes there are three cultural responses to death which he defines as traditional, modern and neo-modern (Walter 1994). These represent the three contexts of a trajectory of dying, which are the bodily, social and authority contexts (Walter 1994; Auger 2007). The dying trajectory following withdrawal of treatment in the ICU may be perceived as modern, hidden and controlled. Aries (1974) suggests the emerging attitude towards death in the twentieth century is one of death denial or invisible death where most people die in hospitals rather than at home (Auger 2007). The dying person is removed from the community, dying and death are hidden, and the care of the dead moves from the private realm of the home to the public domain of healthcare professionals and the hospital environment (Aries 1974; Auger 2007). This concept of hidden death is especially apt with regards to the dying patient undergoing withdrawal of treatment in the CCU.

Glaser & Strauss (1965; 1964) and Sudnow (1967) conducted studies that reflect the ways in which social death is accomplished in acute hospital settings. Sudnow's (1967) research concerns the social action of dying and argues that dying places a frame of interpretation around people resulting in social death practices that serve to isolate them. Aries (1974) states this is the general attitude of western societies towards death, which is characterised by fear and shame. The inherent complexities of the CCU create a problem for dying patients. However, maintaining privacy for the patient and family during the dying trajectory following withdrawal of treatment poses challenges for nurses due to the busyness of the CCU. The closure of curtains around the patient's bed space serves symbolically as a 'traffic light' system with regards to dignity and respect during the patient's dying.

Sudnow (1967) and Glaser & Strauss (1965) describe how nurses and doctors practise avoidance of the dying situation through pretending to deliver information and attention to routine tasks. Sudnow (1967) supports the notion that the associated meanings pertinent to the dying process and death are the product of social interaction. Dying is socially defined by doctors and nurses in that the actual moment of biological death becomes temporally dissociated from the moment of social death, and as a result the patient is treated and perceived as if biological death has already occurred (Sudnow 1967).

Auger (2007) suggests biological death is determined to some extent by medical technology, whereas social death remains difficult to define because individuals are not always aware of its occurrence in their lives. Glaser & Strauss (1965) explored the question of whether people could die socially before they died biologically and what this meant for human relationships. In 1965, Glaser and Strauss published *Awareness of Dying*, and uncovered a social process termed 'awareness contexts'. Critical to their theory was the recognition that dying is a social process that occurs over time. Critically ill sedated patients are usually unaware of their impending death which may be interpreted as 'closed' awareness, whereas the patient's family experience 'open' awareness towards the patient's dying trajectory through discussion and explanation with critical care practitioners. Nurses maintain professional composure by managing their emotional involvement with the patient according to their expectations regarding the patient's death (Goopy 2006). The intensity of critical caring helps to take a nurse's mind off the patient's fate, thus reducing the nurse's conscious involvement and helps in maintaining composure during this fraught and fragile time of withdrawal of treatment (Goopy 2006). Additionally, nurses rely on each other for mutual support to maintain their composure and to be reassured that everything conceivable has been done for the patient.

Unnecessary suffering and ineffective communication at end-of-life in the CCU is thought to be due to the difficulty of identifying the perfect time to implement the shift from a cure focus to comfort care (Efstathiou & Clifford 2011). Providing end-of-life care following cessation of treatment is further complicated because of the short duration of the patient's dying phase. The risk of a sudden imminent death does not allow for preparation for death as it places enormous demands and challenges on the nurses, who are expected to deliver high-quality end-of-life care for the dying patient and bereaved family in a very short time (Morgan 2008).

Viewing death as a failure

Understanding the role of embodiment in social life requires recognition that our bodies give us both life and death, so that social and cultural life can be understood as a human construction in the face of death (Seale 1998). Furthermore, the critical care culture is primarily one of using advanced technology to save lives and increase the patient's chances of survival. For many nurses, discussions relevant to dying and death appear difficult in this technologically proactive care setting where practitioners may feel that a patient's death reflects poorly on their skills and represents a failure on their part to save the patient's life (Curtis & Patrick 2001). Discomfort in discussing death appears to be universal and not a problem unique to critical care nurses alone, as it is rooted in society's denial of dying and death (Curtis & Patrick, 2001).

Critically ill, sedated patients who undergo mechanical ventilation with an artificial airway in situ are usually unable to communicate verbally due to their unconscious and aphonic state. There is a close connection between the nurse and a patient through the immediacy of the body and the gaze (Vouzavali et al. 2011). Although sedated and ventilated, these patients are arousable from their sedated state by manipulating the dosage of the sedative infusion. However, in some patients who are in a haemodynamically labile state this may not be possible. Cirlot (1995) affirms that 'watching' is symbolic of understanding, while 'gaze' symbolises the development of empathy. The nurse and patient reveal themselves through their eye contact, a mutual gaze that encompasses each other's world, care and intimacy with the eyes symbolising the path to the body and the soul.

Through the body a relationship develops between a patient and a nurse (Vouzavali et al. 2011). Additionally, the continuity of care and a nurse/patient ratio of 1:1 provide an ideal opportunity for the development of an intimate relationship between the nurse and a patient. Through this mutual gaze a deeper communication and understanding are achieved, a bond develops when oral communication is not possible, and empathy is mediated by the mere sight of and contact with a patient's body and often their gaze (Vouzavali et al. 2011). The intensive care nurse develops a close relationship with the critically ill sedated patient by collating information pertinent to the patient's disease entities, individual assessment of holistic needs, treatment profile, case notes and explanations from the family.

Fisher (2001) explained that the success of intensive care was not to be measured only by survival statistics, as though each death was a medical failure; instead it should be measured by the quality of lives preserved or restored, the quality of those dying and the quality of relationships involved in each death. Despite the best intentions of intensive care staff to provide more humane and compassionate end-of-life care, the prospect of dying and death, along with the silence that punctuates a family discussion about death and the feeling of desolation and hopelessness that death evokes, still induces a degree of physical and emotional discomfort (Levy 2001).

The use of technological life support creates an interlude during which people strive to harmonise their understandings, expectations and plans for the patient (Cook 2001). Family members often need time to overcome denial that the patient is dying and disbelief that treatment options no longer exist, or to restore healthy family dynamics. Early on during the patient's CCU journey, technological support is collectively viewed by the patient's family as saving life and 'doing everything', rather than as specific technological tools with specific therapeutic uses, thus representing a global approach to achieving the goals of care (Pattison 2011). During the withdrawal process, the use of this technology could be viewed by the family as 'stopping everything', which may appear upsetting and undignified, as the goal of technology thus appears to shift from saving life to inducing pain or prolonging death.

The stage is the critical care unit where the scene is set around an unconscious, critically ill patient who no longer responds to maximum biotechnological live-sustaining supportive therapies. Closed curtains shelter the vulnerable patient from the rest of the critical care milieu and the patient's bed space serves as a protected and private area where dying and death will ensue. There are different players enacting their respective roles as doctors, nurses and family members. The patient is silent due to a sedative and analgesic induced state. Once the decision to withdraw treatment has been made, the family's attendance at a meeting is requested and the family are notified of the decision. The nurse will prepare the setting and patient, create an appropriate environment for dying, and support the family as the withdrawal of treatment unfolds. This close, intimate relationship of mutual trust and respect between a silent patient, nurse and the family are integral to this dying journey to death following the decision to withdraw life-sustaining therapies from the critically ill patient.

This is the surreal life world of the practitioners who work in the CCU, where death appears often but dying is constant. The following scenario describes the timeline of a withdrawal of treatment process from field notes during the observational phase of my doctoral research.

Withdrawal of treatment: observations and field notes (Templeman 2015)

The scene setting – despite maximum medical therapy and technological supportive therapy for multiple organ failure, the patient's condition has steadily deteriorated rather than improving, and has not responded to the supportive therapy administered. The secretary explains that each patient's vital signs are apparent on the central computer at the nurses' station. I am impressed by her knowledge and insight as she explains what each continuous tracing and value signifies and appears to have insight as to what is normal and what is abnormal. These rows of luminous green numerical values and tracings for each patient cascade across the monitor screen highlighting a life which exists beyond this myriad of wires, tubes and machinery attached to the patient. The identical tracings and values are reflected on the monitor above the patient's bed space.

Curtain close – the curtain is drawn around the patient's bed space which the nurse tells me is to maintain patient privacy, especially when the staff are working with the patient or assessing the patient. A constant hissing and clicking sound is audible from the patient's bed space. The nurse informs me that these sounds are coming from the mechanical ventilator and the renal haemofiltration machine.

Decision making – the curtain is drawn around the patient's bed space and a flurry of voices may be heard from behind the curtain now. This is followed by a discussion which takes place at the foot of the patient's bed but outside the curtain, involving all the staff present. The nurse caring for this patient and the ICU secretary are my key informants on this particular day of observation. I later learn from the nurse that the discussion which occurred at the foot of the bed involved the team discussing the ethical and moral issues, physiological indicators, current clinical profile and prognosis pertinent to the patient, and the rationale for not escalating or continuing further treatment. Although the discussion occurs in low voice tones, it is still audible. It is apparent that the intensive care personnel are actively contributing towards and are engaged in the debate and discussion. The team then enter the patient's bed space behind the closed curtain again, but further discussion is no longer audible. The team emerge from behind the closed curtain, which is drawn back slightly by the nurse caring for the patient, and the consultant busily writes on the documents at the foot of the bed.

The decision is made to withdraw treatment – the morning intensive care assessment round continues as the team then make their way to the next bed space to review the next patient. The nurse informs me, after the team have moved to the next patient's bed space, that the consultant has documented his decision to withdraw treatment for this patient today. She mentions that the consultant is responsible for making the final decision regarding withdrawal of treatment and that it is legally binding to document this decision clearly on the patient's charts. The rationale behind this decision is based on the ethical principle of futility in agreement within the multi-disciplinary critical care team. She then goes about her work in a quiet manner but appears rather subdued and has a sombre look on her face. The decision has been made, and the nurse informs me that she will now notify the patient's family to come in so that the consultant may break the news to them. Next, she will prepare the patient and the bed space (i.e. remove all unnecessary equipment from the bed area) for the impending withdrawal of treatment.

The beginning of the end – in contrast to the hive of nursing and medical activity prior to the morning round, there appears now to be a sudden lull and quietness surrounding the patient's bed space, after the team continue with the intensive care morning round. The mood throughout the CCU appears sombre; even the CCU secretary is less talkative. It is somehow apparent that the rest of the personnel are aware of the impending withdrawal of treatment from this patient. The nurse walks over to the nurses' station and conducts a telephonic conversation with the family of the patient, informing them that their presence is requested in the CCU. She returns to the patient's bed space and spends some time talking to the nurse in the adjacent bed space. The secretary tells me she is 'handing the patient over' and the other nurse 'will keep an eye' on her patient while she has her morning break. The nurse then exits the unit for her morning break. After a while, she returns from her break and closes the curtain, with another nurse in attendance. Their voices may be heard behind the closed curtain and it appears that they are explaining things to the patient. The second nurse exits the bed space carrying what appears to be soiled bed linen. The patient's nurse emerges several times after this, collects two blue plastic chairs and enters behind the closed curtains. A little later, she collates some paperwork from the nurses' station which she takes with her to the patient's bed space.

Arrival of patient's family – the curtain surrounding the bed space will remain closed throughout the procedure of withdrawal of treatment and the patient's subsequent dying trajectory.

After about an hour, the front door buzzer of the CCU heralds the arrival of the patient's family. The CCU secretary goes over to the nurse behind the curtain and quietly announces that the relatives of the patient have arrived. The relatives (a middle-aged man and woman) hurriedly enter the CCU and appear nervous. They are greeted by the nurse at the patient's bed space. She speaks to them in a caring and friendly manner, ushering them into the bed space behind the closed curtain. After a while she emerges and disappears for a few minutes, and on her return is followed by the consultant.

You are not alone – together they usher the relatives out of the CCU. The secretary informs me they have been taken to the private counselling room within the CCU complex where the news is broken regarding the decision to withdraw treatment and the patient's impending death is discussed. The consultant, the nurse and the relatives return to the patient bed space once again, where the consultant proceeds to join the multi-disciplinary team on the CCU round. The female relative is supported by the nurse who links her arm into the relative's arm. They are behind the closed curtain again. Soft crying and muffled voices are audible from the patient's bed space.

The dying trajectory unfolds – this scenario of soft crying and muffled voices continues for the next hour. No one leaves the bed space during this time. The nurse stays with the relatives at the patient's bedside throughout this time behind the closed curtain. Only the hiss of the ventilator is audible. I glance at the monitor screen at the nurses' station and notice that the patient's numerical values have decreased, especially her heart rate. The rest of the CCU personnel continue with what appears to be their normal daily activities with the occasional bonging of alarms, telephones ringing at the nurses' station, and the CCU entrance buzzer heralding the arrival of internal and external visitors. Throughout the withdrawal of treatment, there is a steady flow of people entering and leaving the unit, some with stethoscopes hung around their necks but all dressed in plain clothes. Several trolleys are wheeled into the CCU, some heavily laden with linen stacked high, and others with a multitude of boxes varying in size which I am told is pharmacy and general stock replacement. However, the noise level throughout the CCU appears quieter. Behind the closed curtain, silence reigns at the patient's bed space and very little movement is apparent. The relatives' sobbing and voices talking in a low tone are now barely audible from behind the curtain. The decreasing numerical values on the nurses' station monitor reflect the unfolding scene which is taking place behind the closed curtain, signifying the patient's dying trajectory. I notice that as the patient's heart rate slows down, the louder the sobbing behind the curtains becomes. The nurse's voice is audible at the start of the withdrawal of treatment, but her tone now appears softer as the patient's heart rate drops.

The patient dies – suddenly the hissing noise stops, the crying is now audibly louder at the bedside for a short period of time and then there is silence. A few minutes later the sobbing relatives emerge from behind the closed curtain followed closely by the nurse, and together they exit the CCU. The nurse returns to the CCU after about 15 minutes and notifies the anaesthetic registrar of the patient's death. He then enters the patient's bed space to certify the patient's death. This is later confirmed by the nurse when I enquire about it. The relatives of the deceased patient do not come back into the CCU.

Curtains open – the curtain is only opened again after the nurse and another nurse have conducted the last offices and the patient's body is removed to the hospital mortuary. The nurse takes a break for 45 minutes in the staff tea room. I join the nurse in the staff tea room for my break where she remarks:

> *well, we did everything in our power to sustain the patient's life. But unfortunately it was not good enough! … anyway at least we could ensure a dignified and pain free death for the patient! It is just so hard for the relatives you know … knowing there is nothing more we can do for the patient. I feel very sad when we withdraw treatment and sometimes it is difficult to not cry when you are with the relatives and everyone involved with the care of the patient feels a sense of helplessness and loss*

Reflections of a chapter of life fully spent in ICU – the nurse explains her role during withdrawal of treatment and the patient's dying trajectory to me. She mentions her remit involves supporting the family and to ensure the patient is comfortable, pain free and has a dignified death. Once the consultant has confirmed and documented the withdrawal of treatment, the nurse caring for the patient prepares for and conducts the withdrawal of treatment. This is a nurse-led practice whereby the nurse's role is heightened by living the experience with the patient and the family, supporting them whilst also conducting the withdrawal of treatment. We sip our coffee in silence, while I write my notes and the nurse blankly pages through a magazine and occasionally directs her attention to the plasma television screen on the wall. I ask her if she would like to talk about her feelings regarding the withdrawal of treatment, but she tearfully declines, saying:

> *aw, it is just nice to be here* [in the tea room] *away from it all for a while, I know you know what it is like, sometimes it helps just to know someone understands what we intensive care nurses go through.*

And life continues – the nurse enters the unit again from her break and helps another nurse with a new admission, a patient who has arrived from the recovery room. She disappears behind the curtain drawn behind the patient's bed space. From the time the multi-disciplinary team leave the patient's bed area, the following two hours and 40 minutes of events appear to be time-lapsed in an unknown yet shared transitional journey. (***Extracts from field notes***.)

The patient's dying journey to death has unfolded and shifted from a curative, rescue focus to an end-of-life perspective – from a life event which encompasses technological and advanced supportive measures to sustain life at all costs, to attempting to mimic natural dying, an (un)certain death at an unknown time. A patient has died, a family and a nurse face their separate bereaved states and life continues in the ever-changing world of the CCU.

Conclusion

This chapter has offered a unique insight into a cultural environment where life and death is played out on a daily basis. Of course this is but one 'snapshot' in time through an anthropological lens. I would like to share with you at this point some of the overall findings of the ethnographic research, so that what you have read above is seen in the overall interpretation of other cultural themes:

Three central themes emerged from the data analysis, namely: the decision to withdraw treatment; nurses' actions following the withdrawal of treatment decision; and shared experiences in the journey towards death. The findings suggested that nurses' created a private space for the dying patient and discovered a parallel journey towards death experienced by the patient, the nurse and the family. The nurse's adaptation from a curative focus of care to palliative care also emerged, where the desire was to offer positive and meaningful experiences for the family during this emotive phase of 'end-of-life care'. Recommendations for clinical practice include the recognition of the value and benefits of formal and informal support for nurses during the patient's withdrawal of treatment and subsequent dying trajectory. Recognition of the importance of the intensive care environment as a whole for dying patients, their families and their care cannot be undervalued. In addition, given the palliative nature of care required of critical care nurses, a recommended inclusion of a palliative care specialist nurse in the multi-disciplinary team could enhance the patients' quality of end-of-life care. (Abstract: Templeman 2015)

References

Aries P (1974) *Western Attitudes Towards Death: From the Middle Ages to the Present*, Johns Hopkins University Press, London.
Auger J A (2007) *Social Perspectives on Death and Dying*, 2nd Edition, Fernwood Publishing, Canada.
Bryan L (2007) Should ward nurses hide death from other patients? *End of Life Care*, 1(1), 79–86.
Callahan D (1995) *The Troubled Dream of Life*, Touchstone, New York.
Chambers N & Curtis J R (2001) The interface of technology and spirituality in the ICU. In J R Curtis & G D Rubenfeld (eds), *Managing Death in the Intensive Care Unit: The Transition from Cure to Comfort*, Oxford University Press, New York.
Cirlot J E (1995) *A Dictionary of Symbols*, Konidaris, Athens.
Cook D (2001) Patient autonomy versus parentalism, *Critical Care Medicine*, 29(2), N24–N25. Coombs M A, Long-Sutehall T & Shannon S (2010) International dialogue on end of life challenges in the UK and USA, *Journal of British Association of Critical Care Nurses* , 15(5), 234–240.
Coombs M A, Addington-Hall J & Long-Sutehall T (2011) Challenges in transition from intervention to end of life care in intensive care: A qualitative study, *International Journal of Nursing Studies*, 49, 519–527.
Costello J (2006) Dying well: Nurses' experiences of 'good and bad' deaths in hospital, *Issues and Innovation in Nursing Practice*, 594–601.
Curtis R J & Patrick D L (2001) The role of quality of life and health status in making decisions about withdrawing life-sustaining treatments in the ICU. In R J Curtis & G D Rubenfeld (eds), Managing Death in the Intensive Care Unit: The Transition from Cure to Comfort, Oxford University Press, New York.
Cypress B S (2011) The lived ICU experience of nurses, patients and family members: A phenomenological study with Merleau-Pontian perspective, *Intensive and Critical Care Nursing*, 1–8.
Efstathiou N & Clifford C (2011) The critical care nurse's role in end-of-life care: Issues and challenges, *British Association of Critical Care Nurses: Nursing in Critical Care*, 16(3), 116–123.
Glaser B G & Strauss A L (1964) The social loss of dying patients, *The American Journal of Nursing*, 4(6), 119–121.
Glaser B G & Strauss A L (1965) *Awareness of Dying*, Aldine, Chicago.
Goopy S (2006) … that the social order prevails: Death, ritual and the 'Roman' nurse, *Nursing Inquiry*, 3(2), 110–117.

Hallam E & Hockey J (2001) *Death, Memory and Material Culture*, Berg, Oxford.

Hockey J, Komarov C. & Woodthorpe K (2010) *The Matter of Death: Space, Place and Materiality*, Palgrave Macmillan, UK.

Holland C K (1993) An ethnographic study of nursing culture as an exploration for determining the existence of a system of ritual, *Journal of Advanced Nursing*, 18, 1461–1470.

Illich I (1976) *Limits to Medicine/Medical Nemesis: The Expropriation of Health*, Penguin Books, London.

Intensive Care Society (ICS) (2009) *Guidelines for Limitation of Treatment for Adults Requiring Intensive Care*, London.

Kirchhoff K T, Spuhler V, Walker L, Hutton A, Cole B V & Clemmer T (2006) Intensive care nurses' experiences with end-of-life care, *American Journal of Critical Care*, 9(1), 36–42.

Latour J M, Fulbrook P and Albarran J W (2009) EfCCNa survey: European intensive care nurses' attitudes and beliefs towards end-of-life care, *Nursing in Critical Care*, 14(3), 110–121.

McMillen R E (2007) End of life decisions: Nurses' perceptions, feelings and experiences, *Intensive and Critical Care Nursing*, 24, 251–259.

Miller P A, Forbes S & Boyle D K (2001) End-of-life in the intensive care unit: A challenge for nurses, *American Journal of Critical Care*, 10(4), 230–237.

Mohammed S & Peter E (2009) Rituals, death and the moral practice of medical futility, *Nursing Ethics*, 16(3), 292–302.

Morgan J (2008) End-of-life care in UK critical care units – A literature review, *British Association of Critical Care Nurses*, 13(3), 152–161.

Olausson S, Ekebergh M & Osterberg S A (2014) Nurses' lived experiences of intensive care unit bed spaces as a place of care: A phenomenological study, *British Association of Critical Care Nurses*, 19(30), 126–133.

Pattison N (2004) Integration of palliative care and critical care at end of life, *British Journal of Nursing*, 13, 132–139.

Pattison N (2011) End of life in critical care: An emphasis on care, *Nursing in Critical Care*, 16(3), 113–115.

Philpin S M (2007) Managing ambiguity and danger in an intensive therapy unit: ritual practices and sequestration, *Nursing Inquiry*, 14(1), 51–59.

Rocker G, Puntillo K A, Azoulay E & Nelson J E (2010) *End of Life Care in the ICU: From Advanced Disease to Bereavement*, Oxford University Press, Oxford.

Seale C (1998) *Constructing Death: The Sociology of Dying and Death*, Cambridge University Press, Cambridge.

Seymour J E (2001) *Critical Moments: Death and Dying in Intensive Care*, Open University Press, Milton Keynes.

Sudnow D (1967) *Passing on*, Prentice-Hall, New York.

Suominen T, Kovasim M & Ketola O (1997) Nursing culture – some viewpoints, *Journal of Advanced Nursing Studies*, 25, 186–190.

Templeman J (2015) *An ethnographic study of critical care nurses' experiences following the decision to withdraw life-sustaining treatment from patients in a UK intensive care unit*, Unpublished PhD study, University of Salford, Salford.

Turner V (1969) *The Ritual Process: Structure and Anti-Structure*, Aldine, Chicago. Van Gennep A (1909) *Les rites de passage (The Rites of Passage)*, É. Nourry, Paris.

Van Gennep A (2004) *The Rites of Passage*, Routledge, London.

Vouzavali F J D, Papathanassoglou E D E, Karanikola M N K, Koutroubas A, Patiraki E I & Papadatou D (2011) 'The patient is my space': Hermeneutic investigation of the nurse-patient relationship in critical care, *Nursing in Critical Care*, 16(3), 140–151.

Walter T (1994) *The Revival of Death*, Routledge, London.

Further reading

1   AriesP (1981) *The Hour of our Death*, Peregrine Books, London.
2   British Medical Association (2001) *Withholding and Withdrawing Life-Prolonging Medical Treatment*, British Medical Association, London.

3   Ciccarello G P (2003) Strategies to improve end-of-life care in the intensive care unit, *Dimensions of Critical Care Nursing*, 22, 216–222.

4   Cook D, Rocker G, Giacomini M, Sinuff T & Heyland D (2006) Understanding and changing attitudes toward withdrawal and withholding of life support in the intensive care unit, *Critical Care Medicine*, 34(11), 317–323.

5   Crawley I M, Marshall P A, Lo B & Koenig B A (2002) Strategies for culturally effective end-of-life care, *Annals of Internal Medicine*, 136, 673–679.

6   Curtis J R & Rubenfeld G D (2001) *Managing death in the Intensive Care Unit – The Transition from Cure to Comfort*, Oxford University Press, Oxford.

7   Geertz C (1973) *The Interpretation of Cultures*, Basic Books, New York.

8   Hockey J (1990) *Experiences of Death: An Anthropological Account*, Edinburgh University Press, Edinburgh.

9   Nelson J E (2010) *End of Life Care in the ICU: From Advanced Disease to Bereavement*, Oxford University Press, Oxford.

10 Pattison N (2006) A critical discourse analysis of provision of end-of-life care in key UK critical care documents, *British Association of Critical Care Nurses*, 11(4), 198–208.

11 Philpin S M (2004) *An Interpretation of Ritual and Symbolism in an Intensive Therapy Unit*, Unpublished PhD study, University of Wales Swansea, Swansea.

12 Philpin S M (2006) 'Handing over': Transmission of information between nurses in an intensive therapy unit, *Nursing in Critical Care*, 11(2), 86–93.

13 Robben A C G M (ed) (2009) *Death, Mourning and Burial – A Cross-Cultural Reader*, Blackwell Publishing, Oxford.

14 Templeman J (2015) *An ethnographic study of critical care nurses' experiences following the decision to withdraw life-sustaining treatment from patients in a UK intensive care unit*, Unpublished PhD study, University of Salford, Salford (http://usir.salford.ac.uk/id/eprint/36188/1/Prof%20Doc%20thesis%20(final%20version%202015).pdf).

15 Turner V W (1967) *The Forest of Symbols*, Cornell University Press, New York.

16 Waraporn K (2009) Promoting peaceful death in the intensive care unit in Thailand, *International Nursing Review*, 56(1), 116–122.

17 Zerubavel E (1979) *Patterns of Time in Hospital Life: A Sociological Perspective*, University of Chicago Press, Chicago.

10

NURSING AND CULTURE

Language, knowledge and power

Benny Goodman

Introduction

This chapter draws from the *social* and *cultural* anthropological approach and also from social science theory, especially that of Margaret Archer and Michel Foucault. These ideas will be used to begin a critical reflection on how our *agency*, our *freedom to act*, operates within social *structures* and *cultures*, how language and discourses can create and be created by social realities and 'the self', in their use in everyday practice. I suggest that 'culture flows through self and vice versa'. I also consider how discourses, such as the 'Biomedical', the 'Institutional Psychiatric' and the 'Moral Underclass', might provide the cultural context for nursing actions and knowledge. This includes our decisions about what is the appropriate course to take on, for example, health and social inequalities and our *explanations for* health and social inequalities.

I suggest that we are human agents that pre-exist society but we act within structural and cultural circumstances over time, actions which are mediated by our reflexive deliberations within discourses. However, we are not free 'independent of society' autonomous beings using rational thought to choose courses of action as assumed by many discourses on health behaviour.

It is argued here that many health care professionals are insufficiently aware of how *taken for granted* (cultural) assumptions are built into certain health and illness discourses so that these assumptions become *common sense*. They are also unaware that these assumptions operate in certain social structures, an example of which is the class/command dynamic of neoliberal financial capitalism (Grant & Goodman 2018; Scambler 2012).

This results in, for example, 'lifestyle drift' responses (Hunter et al. 2009) to public health issues such as obesity, and on health inequalities. Lifestyle drift responses often implicitly focus on changing working class culture and using individual behaviour change techniques as *common sense and taken for granted* solutions to *structural* inequalities in health. This lack of awareness is not surprising because health care professionals are educated within the discourses of scientific medicine and not the critical social sciences.

I suggest that if a deeper discussion is wanted, the reader access the work of Margaret Archer (1982; 1988; 1995; 2000; 2008; 2010) which provides the social theory that underpins this tentative exploration of how the relationship between human agency, social structure and culture actually plays out in the world. Foucault's work can be difficult to read especially for those with little social science knowledge. (See Grant & Goodman 2018 for a brief introduction to Foucault's 'discourse'.)

I will begin with a brief overview of what anthropology in nursing might mean before addressing Archer and Foucault's key concepts. I will outline the 'Structure-Agency-Culture' model and the role of Reflexive Deliberations within it, followed by Subject Positioning, Governmentality and finally Discourse. Examples of discourses will be outlined in an attempt to illustrate how the interplay between culture, human agency and structure could be understood by nurses.

Anthropology and the centrality of culture

According to the Royal Anthropological Institute (2017) anthropology:

> is the study of people throughout the world, their evolutionary history, how they behave, adapt to different environments, communicate and socialise with one another. The study of anthropology is concerned both with the biological features that make us human and with social aspects (such as language, culture, politics, family and religion) (my emphasis).

The American Anthropological Association (2017) points out that the discipline, in the USA, draws upon the social and biological sciences to investigate human *cultures* across history. In the USA the discipline subdivides into four areas:

1. sociocultural
2. biological/physical
3. archaeological
4. linguistic.

Engelke (2017a) emphasises the study of *culture* to make the 'familiar strange and the strange familiar' a concern with the 'everyday'. It examines the *taken for granted* everyday aspects of social life as a focus for study and as such shares the approach of Ethnomethodology – the study of 'people's methods' used to make a 'common sense' view of everyday life. Ethnomethodology (Garfinkel 1974) uses 'conversation analysis' to do so. Note: 'Ethnomethodology' (a sociological theory) is not to be confused with 'Ethnography' (a research approach used to study cultural phenomena from the perspective of the subjects of the study) (see Chapter 3).

Placing 'culture' as a central concept, Engelke directs us towards the study of our values, norms, behaviours and language as well as art, music and ritual. Culture is important because it provides the lenses through which we view the world, it is *'the index of our ideas and values and modes of reasoning'*. Culture *'wears the garb of common sense'* (Engelke 2017b).

This idea of 'common sense' is really important as it is often implicitly invoked when considering courses of action on for example 'obesity', as seen in the injunctions to 'eat less – move more'. These 'common sense' understandings can build into a 'common sense' discourse on health, one that often places the blame for illness, or weight gain, firmly onto the individual's shoulders due to their poor lifestyle choices.

In Chapter 1, Karen Holland provides three definitions of anthropology for consideration, an established one, from medical anthropology and two possible ones for an anthropology of nursing. Again core concepts include *culture* but importantly as it operates within a social and temporal context. In this chapter, I'd like to add a further consideration of the interplay between structure, agency and culture to understand nursing work at this point in history.

Margaret Archer (1995) has argued that we need to be more analytically precise in conceptualising 'culture' and its place in human affairs. In her Morphogenetic approach, outlined in her 'trilogy' (Archer 2003; 2007; 2012), we are asked to think about human agency in the context of social *structure* and *culture* and how reflexivity (our inner conversations) mediates the relationship between objective social conditions and our human agency.

In other words: this is about 'human agency' (Marx's: *'we make our own history'*) and structural and cultural circumstances (*'but not in the circumstances of our own making'*). Human beings cannot be reduced to social and cultural constructs or emerge as products of language, but the complete freedom to think and act may be more complicated than adherents of the *'autonomous sovereign individual of the liberal human self'* (Grant & Goodman 2018) of modernity may have us believe.

Archer (2000) describes this 'man of modernity' arising out of Enlightenment thinking as *'a being whose fundamental constitution owes nothing to society'* (p. 51) and increasingly driven by instrumental rationality. This is the 'ready-made man' who turns up out of nowhere to impose his own order on the world and applies rational thought to social concerns. It is a view of 'self' that is ontologically separate from society, not constituted at all by society or culture, but is an independent free thinking and rational being. Nurses will hear echoes of this 'man's' voice when they hear such statements as *'only the individual should and can take responsibility for health'*, *'there is no such thing as society, just individuals and families'*.

There is not the space to *fully* explore this idea of the 'free, pre-existing, independent from society' view of self, other than to suggest that extricating human agency and the 'self' completely out of the effects of culture and social structure is erroneous.

The reason for this will be covered in the next section. I emphasise, however, the pernicious persistence of this idea in current culture and its underpinning for understanding human behaviour towards health. I take the view that culture flows through self and both *constitutes* and is *constituted by* self but without fully dissolving the notion of a self into society or culture so that 'the self' completely disappears into either.

Understanding structure, agency and culture

Graham Scambler (2013d), in wishing to establish a theory of agency in sociology, argues: *'Humans … are simultaneously the products of biological, psychological and social mechanisms while retaining their agency … socially structured without being structurally determined'* (p. 147).

Who, and what, we are arises socially, as well as from our physical biological selves, as well as from our psychological thinking and motivations.

Social structures are institutional systems or patterns of human interaction which help to organise and give meaning to society. *Class* structures are often identified by socio-economic status as outlined in the NS-SEC classification. Examples of a *family* structure are the nuclear family or the extended family. *Occupational* structures in hospitals include multi-professional teams and management hierarchies. Structures have heterogeneous *cultures*, for example a *white British* nuclear family *structure* might exhibit very different cultural traits (their food choices, family values, dress) than a *black or minority ethnic* nuclear family. The structure is the same (nuclear family) but the culture varies.

Society *structures* who we are without *determining* who we are. We are born into a class structure, an ethnic structure, gender structures, a family structure, and have opportunities to join certain occupational structures. The family you are born into – i.e. its place in the class structure – will highly structure your future choices and opportunities. That's why we see middle class families being over-represented in certain schools, universities and occupations.

Family life structures us – providing language, values, customs, hopes and aspirations – but does not *determine* these aspects of ourselves. In the same way, socio-economic and class structures are also contexts in which our agency operates. The very way you speak is often a construct of your social class background. The fact that the nursing profession is a female gendered structure reflects how our choices are being 'structured'.

Medicine, traditionally male, and still so at the senior consultant level, reflects similar structural effects on the human (agential) choices of career. In addition, the (female, caring, nurturing) *culture* of certain professions, however, may make it easier or harder for (male) free agents to want to exercise those choices. Culture thus interplays with structure and agency.

Agency: There is room for *agency – the freedom to act as an agent*; the freedom for men to choose nursing despite social structures and cultures of nursing. A clinical setting structures us and provides a culture – giving us a language, a discourse, acceptable modes of professional behaviours and explicit values, but it does not *determine* who we are as professionals. (See Chapter 8 for issues related to men in nursing as a choice.)

Culture: The everyday aspects of social life, the taken for granted common sense practices, assumptions and values shared within a social group expressed in their behaviours and attitudes. Examples of culture are myriad. The fondness of British people for a 'nice cup of tea' is culture. Nursing culture may include 'coping under pressure' which manifests as working longer hours than contracted for. (See Chapter 2 for alternatives.)

George Orwell (1941) described English cultural traits such as a 'love of flowers' and 'addictions to hobbies'. He suggested that the English were not puritanical as we were inveterate gamblers, beer drinkers, lovers of bawdy jokes and use the foulest language in the world! Consider if we can agree what English culture is today.

Structure and Culture are the contexts for Agency. How free agents choose courses of action within cultures and structures is discussed at length by Margaret Archer using her notion of 'modes of reflexivity'. Archer (2010) argues that: '*reflexivity mediates between the objective structural and cultural contexts confronting agents, who activate their properties as constraints and enablements as they pursue reflexively defined "projects" based on their concerns*' (p. 1).

The way a health care professional *thinks* about a course of action in any given clinical context will be manifest in what they do, what aims they set themselves and will be based in how they see their abilities, options, *enablements and constraints*. They do so in an objective structural and cultural context. The clinic, the ward, the home is the objective setting. What you say and what you do operates there.

However, the model of the 'liberal human self' outlined above assumes the primacy of agency devoid of structure or cultural contexts. Thus we might think that obese and overweight people freely choose to eat more than they need, that their inability to lose weight is down to their weak moral character. They should 'just say no' to a second pork pie.

Against this I suggest that they eat and move within the structure of the '*obesogenic environment*' (Foresight 2007) and within cultural practices around food that become aspects of *who they are*, that they build into their self-concept. Veganism, for example, has been seen as the preserve of a (slightly effete?) minority and for many men especially cannot be built into their own notions of self as 'red meat-eating masculinity'. Their self-concept as a man excludes this food choice as viable. They are of course free to act as a vegan but the structural and cultural context militates against many men doing so.

In the same way we might think nurses are free to prescribe medications as they choose within the formulary but they do so within certain accepted pharmaceutical frames of reference and medical discourses that steer the decisions towards a drugs-based solution to certain health and social problems. The use of antidepressants is an example of this contested space of appropriate prescribing in which a psychiatric culture clashes with an antipsychiatry culture (Moore 2018).

They are free to prescribe but not in the circumstances of their own choosing. It is to these 'circumstances' (the structural and cultural context) we must look to more fully understand those choices.

Uncritical reflection and a lack of critical reflexivity within certain clinical structures and cultures could result in nurses ('agents') who practice and think along pre-set lines, using habits, tradition, custom and practice and mental short cuts and who talk using cliché, jargon and technical terms in an unthinking manner to produce what Minnich (2017) calls the '*evil of banality*'.

So we need to see that agency (the freedom to act as an agent) works within a context, e.g. a clinical context, in which the social outcome is structured by that context, but *not determined* by it. So to be very clear, Archer (2012) argues agency operates in the following way:

1. **Situation**: The (clinical practice) setting provides the external, objective, situation and cultural context which the 'free agent' is confronted with. The agent does not have a choice about this. The (clinical) setting provides situations of 'constraint' and 'enablements' for the 'agent'.
2. This objective situation operates in relation to concerns and projects.
3. **Concerns and Projects**: The agent who has their own internal, subjective, *concerns and projects* that relate to their personal epistemologies (their ways of knowing – science, artistry, intuition), their ontologies (what they believe exists such as bacteria, viruses or energy fields), their values (sanctity of life for example), their social realities (e.g. the doctor–nurse–management relationship) and cultural practices (e.g. managerial command/control practices, or the 'coping' culture of character-based moral nursing work).
4. **Action**: The action then undertaken by these structured free agents is produced by '**reflexive deliberations**', i.e. **internal conversations**, about the situation and their own concerns and projects.

On point 3, Margaret Archer argues that the interplay between our internal *concerns* and our *situational* social and environmental contexts is shaped by what she calls a 'mode of reflexivity'. A 'mode of reflexivity' is the manner in which we think about our thinking, our 'inner conversations' that then shape our actions.

Nurses wishing to pursue research from an anthropological standpoint may well consider a reflexive methodology, with Alvesson & Skoldberg (2000) offering the view that: '*by a reflective approach we mean that due attention is paid to the interpretative, political and rhetorical nature of empirical research'* (p. vii).

We can consider here what this (Reflexivity) means for a nurse.

Archer (2012) outlines four 'ideal types' of modes of reflexivity:

1. **Meta reflexivity**: Internal conversations critically evaluate previous inner dialogues and are critical about effective action in society; we may then critique whether effective action is possible before we act. This is about self-monitoring, our thinking about how we think, and when dominance results in self-questioning such as 'why did I say that?', 'why am I so reticent to say what I think?' This mode of reflexivity may be what we are calling critical reflexivity. **Values and understanding** are important. The *meta reflexive nurse* might question the routine use of drugs to treat certain conditions, especially mental health conditions, and then seek out alternative therapies. *A meta reflexive nurse* questions all of their decision making and thinking to understand why they think as they do.

2. **Autonomous reflexivity**: Internal conversations are self-contained, leading directly to action; our inner conversation requires no confirmation with others. Here we have a 'lone inner dialogue' which leads directly to action. **Outcomes** or Goals are important. If one has a NICE guideline to follow, then the autonomous reflexive might just 'get on with it'. *An autonomous reflexive nurse* knows what needs to be done, clearly sets on the goal of action and, despite what others might think, gets on and does it.

3. **Communicative reflexivity**: Internal conversations need to be completed by others before they lead to action; *a nurse who predominantly uses communicative reflexivity* will consider what their peers are thinking and will want to act in such a way as to fit in. **Social cohesion** and **consensus** is important. Again the social safety of a clinical guideline or the custom and practice of peers might not lead to critical examination of the course of action.

4. **Fractured reflexivity**: Internal conversations cannot lead to purposeful action but intensify personal distress and disorientation resulting in expressive action. I would argue here that survival is important. This nurse should not be talking to patients and deciding on treatment options.

Scambler (2013a; 2013b; 2013c) further develops this typology as:

a   Focused Autonomous reflexives.
b   Dedicated Meta reflexives.
c   Vulnerable Fractured reflexives.

So, according to Archer, we have internal conversations. Our inner speech is rapid and often contracted into single words or phrases that contain a rich complexity of meaning. What we then need to consider is how these 'inner conversations' operate in certain structures and cultures.

We might suggest that certain medical and patriarchal cultures and their associated discourses impact on how nurses think about themselves and the course of action they might take, and thus how the culture, expressed though a discourse can *position* nurses and patients into either subservient or equal 'subject positions'.

Subject positioning of nurses and patients

Power and hierarchical cultural contexts based on medical knowledge, managerial and gender roles and expressed through discourses, can empower or disempower nurses and patients as they react to their objective situation. Those nurses and patients who have a dominant mode of '*autonomous reflexivity*' may have the confidence to speak out and act to rebut the positioning by more powerful others. They could be helped in this by establishing new cultures such as 'Family Centred care' or a 'Patient Centred NHS'. The issue of graduate status for student nurses and the continuing arguments over its usefulness in the UK, illustrates a clash of cultures (traditional apprenticeship training v. degree education) that can position some students as 'too posh to wash', a phrase that helps to create discourse and culture of anti-intellectualism in nursing.

According to Davies & Harre (1990) 'positioning' is:

> the discursive process whereby selves are located in conversations as observably and subjectively coherent participants in jointly produced story lines. There can be interactive positioning in which what one person says positions another. And there can be reflexive positioning in which one positions oneself (p. 48).

Note that selves are '*located in* conversations'. It suggests that the words, phrases, sentences you use to another person *puts them in place* to define who they are at that moment. Of course, the other (autonomous reflexive?) person can accept that position or reject it and through language try to claim a different status.

We also use larger discursive *frames* which also position who we think we are and what we think the proper course of action should be.

Consider what nursing frames of reference might be and the degree to which nurses 'borrow' medical frames of reference.

George Lakoff (2004) illustrated 'Framing' as part of political discourse. An example of frames are 'Take Back Control' turning the EU argument into one of sovereignty, the 'War on Drugs' turning substance use into a criminal justice issue rather than a public health issue. You can frame tax as either 'vital investment' or 'theft' depending on your socialist or libertarian leanings.

'Too Posh to Wash' frames nursing as a vocation for which graduate training is not required. Nurses have been framed in the past as self-sacrificial 'Angels'.

We can frame Public Health within a biomedical frame (e.g. vaccinations), or a sanitation frame (the provision of clean water and sewage services) or more recently an ecological frame (Planetary Health). Libertarians also frame public health as 'nanny state interference'.

Discursive practices: At the one-to-one level of interpersonal communication, we build a sense of who we are, who our 'selves' are partly through that interaction. We learn, use and adopt categories which include some categories and not others. These are often binary such as male/female, father/daughter or nurse/patient. We then engage in 'discursive practices' that allocate meaning to those categories. The self is then positioned in relation to the stories that we use for those categories. Consider the category of 'unpopular patient' or 'frequent flyer'. What stories do we use for those categories and thus how do we position ourselves and the categorised person when using them?

Davies and Harre argue that we recognise ourselves as 'belonging' psychologically *and emotionally* to that position (e.g. the 'good nurse', the 'medical expert') through adopting a commitment to a 'world-view' (e.g. caring, compassionate, courageous) that fits with that membership category. Consider the different world views possible for membership of the category of 'patient' or 'client' and how we might position ourselves *and be positioned* as patients/clients through the discursive practices we experience with professionals. Consider if my dominant mode of reflexivity is that of a 'fractured reflexive', how might that affect the outcome?

The concept of 'positioning' describes a fluid and dynamic sense of the multiple 'selves' or 'identities' one has, and also how these 'are called forth' and/or actively constructed, in conversations between people or in other discursive contexts. A GP or Nurse Practitioner consultation is a discursive context mediated by the patient's mode of reflexivity (autonomous, communicative, meta or fractured) within the object cultural context of that consultation (for example the binary positions of 'expert professional – ignorant patient' or 'expert patient – ignorant professional').

How the professional speaks can 'call forth' or deny the patient's expertise and experience and vice versa. The autonomous reflexive patient, however, might resist any other position except themselves as expert.

Sundin-Huard (2001) describes a case study (in the UK) in which the interaction between a nurse and a doctor over the care of a baby, clarified the power dynamic, mutual expectations and discourses available to each of them. The case clearly demonstrated how the nurse was positioned by the discursive practice of the doctor, in that instance, into a passive, submissive role. They had different views of what the baby needed, but the language used by the doctor enabled him to position himself as the more powerful, taking the subject position of 'scientific medical expert'. The nurse's language could not match it, and so she took up the subservient 'handmaiden' subject position resulting in dissonance and frustration.

The nurse began to think of herself, at that moment, as less worthy/powerful than the other. Although now dated, this provided some evidence that suggested nurses had difficulties in making autonomous decisions and/or had problems with their relationships with medical staff.

This is not to suggest, however, that we are passive dupes in such positioning. As argued, we engage in reflexive deliberations which mediate our objective social conditions, our culture and the exercise of our personal agency. In the next section I return to the idea of a discourse in more detail as an aspect of that cultural and structural context. A reminder here is that discourses can become common sense and taken for granted and used to build a sense of one's professional self-identity.

Discourse

In common understanding a 'discourse' is an exchange, perhaps of ideas, between two people involving language as the medium of transmission. This can be seen as a neutral exercise between two people of equal power and status using certain phrases, words, jargon and syntax to share understanding or to question the other's statements. Consider the situation when two health care professionals are talking to each other about a patient's 'prognosis' or 'treatment' and, in an acute medical ward setting, this may take the form of a *biomedical* discourse as the words 'prognosis' and 'treatment' are core words within biomedicine. When one of them then talks to the 'patient', a different 'discourse' may be used in which 'prognosis' is not used in the conversation. At that point the professional has a choice to make: stay within a medical discourse, use lay discourse, or mix them up.

Discourse as a critical concept is associated with Michel Foucault. For Foucault (1969) discourses are *institutionalised* patterns of speech and knowledge seen and felt in 'disciplinary' structures, for example in the medical clinic or in the prison (Foucault 1963; 1969; 1975). Discourses connect knowledge to power, as knowledge *is* power. To oversimplify, the concept refers to the idea that a discourse shapes, or constructs *what and how* we know (epistemology), *what* we can say, and *how* we can say it. The use of the discourse of scientific medicine gives health professionals power over lay persons and policy makers through their access to concepts of the body and treatment options. The discourse of Institutional Psychiatry provides the same power, criticised for the framing of mental distress as a problem within the individual (Grant 2015; Smith & Grant 2016).

The language of medicine in this sense creates a reality in which personal feelings of illness are turned into diagnostic categories expressed in physiological and anatomical terms backed up by disease categories. Those who do not have access to this medical technical language also do not have access to this new reality and are thus in a subordinate less powerful position to those who do. Professionals can use language on others, to *position* them in either equal or subordinate positions using these discourses.

Language can also create a sense of self, who we think we are, and can create a status. Consider the language around a long-term condition such as diabetes. Terms such as Insulin resistance, glycaemic control, blood glucose, metformin, Type 2, glycaemic index, and metabolic syndrome can all be used to create a new sense of self as a 'diabetic'. We may then by adopting such language *position* ourselves in relation to a health professional by speaking on their terms and thus demanding equality. The therapeutic culture can either encourage or dissuade this development in people depending on the values and assumptions (Archer's 'projects and concerns') of the professional engaging with people. This is why talk of changing cultures of care is so prevalent. It is an attempt to equalise and *position* the professional–patient relationship within a non-hierarchical culture.

Discourses are more than mere words. A discourse, Foucault (1969) suggested, actually *brings into being that of which it speaks*:

> discourses … are not … a mere intersection of things and words …. a task that consists of not – of no longer – treating discourses as groups of signs … but as *practices* that systematically **form the objects of which they speak** …. discourses are composed of signs; but what they do is more than use signs to designate things. It is this *more* that renders them irreducible to language and to speech. It is this 'more' that we must reveal and describe (p. 49).

It is as if Foucault is saying that 'objects' do not exist for us until a discourse brings them into existence for us. 'Object' does not refer here always and only to a physical material thing, objects may be abstract concepts such as 'Hypertension' or 'Schizophrenia'. These are words, signs, pointing us to a facet of our reality (the pressure of a fluid in a blood vessel or delusional thoughts) but they are *more* than that.

The word 'Hypertension' is part of the discourse and practice of biomedicine that *creates* a reality for us. Without that discourse describing the pressure of blood in a cardiovascular system, 'hypertension' would not exist. The physical reality of blood circulating and exerting pressure keeping us alive is of course not negated by our lack of knowledge of it. This is so taken for granted by us now because we have been immersed in this discourse; it has been part of our reality for over two centuries. 'Hypertension' exists only because we have that discourse at this time and in certain places especially in critical care units and acute hospitals. It exists only because in *using that word we bring it into existence*. It might be fair to speculate that for Indigenous peoples in the Amazon, isolated from 'civilised' societies, and recourse to biomedical discursive practice, 'hypertension' *does not exist* even if blood circulating obviously still does.

The clearest examples many professionals will hear in their daily work is the 'biomedical discourse' (Jones 1994) or the 'institutional psychiatric discourse' (see Grant 2015; Smith & Grant 2016), both of which use phrases unintelligible to most people. Students actively attend to this new language in their attempts to create a new professional identity, substituting words like cardiac for heart, gastric for tummy and neurological for nerves. In the institutional psychiatric discourse, 'bi-polar' is substituted for the lay term 'manic-depressive', and 'schizophrenia' for 'mad'. Nurse educators actively encourage the adoption of this and other discourses.

The vast gulf that can exist between lay and expert 'epistemology' and 'ontology' of the body can be illustrated by the story of the meaning of the word 'local' as in 'local anaesthetic'. A 28-year-old male was to undergo a simple procedure: a vasectomy. He was told that this was to be performed 'under a local' and consent was sought and given. Not until his arrival in the theatre did the full realisation of what 'local' actually meant sink in. To his mounting anxiety, he realised that in fact the needle was not going to be placed in his gums but somewhere more 'sensitive'. On reflection this was obvious, but why did this not occur to him before?

The health professional gaining consent knows about the central nervous system and peripheral sensory and motor nerves. They know that injecting a drug into a certain anatomical location will provide anaesthesia. They know what a body is. The patient in this scenario had no knowledge of either. His epistemology excluded the physiology of the nervous system and pain pathways. His ontology excluded any knowledge of what the body is in its corporeal form. His only experience of a 'local' was as a child in the dentist's chair having an injection into his gums. 'Local' and 'Gums' were thus inextricably linked and cemented into his epistemology. There was no need to think beyond this accepted use of the word 'local'. So, during the consent period the nurse said 'local' and the patient heard 'local' but what they knew about it varied widely.

This example is perhaps a minor one as the result was the momentary realisation and anxiety in the theatre which meant adjusting to a new reality for the patient. However, it may not take too much thinking to consider how lay and expert epistemologies and ontologies expressed through language can position people into unequal power relationships that have much more far-reaching consequences, especially in the domains of ethical practice, mental health, learning disabilities, public health and critical care.

To further see and feel how knowledge is connected to power, and to understand what is brought into existence by words, I argue that the introduction, implementation, discussion and use of the UK's Chief Nursing Officer's '6Cs' is a newer version of a much older nursing discourse that emphasises the moral and virtuous and perhaps self-sacrificial character of nursing work. (See NHS England website for further information and publications regarding the 6Cs in regards to future 'values based' change in nursing, midwifery and care staff practice: https://www.england.nhs.uk/leadingchange/about/the-6cs/.)

The 6Cs can be seen as a largely uncritically accepted and taken for granted (common sense) discourse with knowledge/power effects. It has been allied to something called 'values based recruitment' in an overt attempt to police those entrants who wish to enter into nursing. The 6Cs and values based recruitment has a language, key words, phrases and action which function in a disciplinary fashion in that they set a boundary within which individual nurses should work, a transgression of which not only could lead to loss of registration but also of moral character and professional identity.

The 6Cs have this primary function of setting out the boundaries of professional nursing practice. They then have a secondary function of policing and protecting professional identity in the face of multiple public criticisms in recent years. The point here is not necessarily whether this is a good or bad thing, rather it is to illustrate how a discourse attempts to shape not only behaviour but how nurses, and others, see and police themselves. The 6Cs is an attempt to change the culture of nursing by building them into the nurses self-concept; in this manner to *be* the 6Cs is *to be* a nurse.

The espoused culture of nursing is to take on the tenets of the 6Cs, a new context in which nursing action should take place and reflect. The *meta reflexive nurse* will think about what that means and if it is possible, the *autonomous reflexive nurse* might accept those as appropriate goals and set them for themselves, *the communicative reflexive nurse* will discuss this and seek consensus on what this means. The *fractured reflexive nurse* will not be able to decide on any course of action.

Using meta reflexivity, I suggest that the discursive practice of using the 6Cs has the surface appearance and function of ensuring 'high-quality patient care based on compassionate practice' as an *espoused theory* but it also has a disciplinary reality aimed at the self-policing by nurses of their own and their colleagues' behaviours as a *theory in action*.

Foucault outlined the concept of 'governmentality' to refer to the idea of self-policing which I would apply to free agents thinking and acting in certain structures and cultures.

Foucault, governmentality and health care culture

Immersion in a culture may act as a 'common sense' guide for practice; the transgression of acceptable cultural practices, and what can be said about that practice, is perhaps policed not just by managers or a hierarchy but by ourselves when we have internalised 'the rules', e.g. the 6Cs, of that culture. As suggested in the next section, if there is a culture that focuses on individual lifestyle explanations for health outcomes, this might over time become the dominant explanation for nurses to use with their patients and with each other. This self-policing is Foucault's 'governmentality'. Governmentality is the process by which power is exercised so that we come to govern *ourselves and each other* without the need to refer to formal authority.

Governmentality is not to be confused with Government. The latter is a top down hierarchical form of power. Governmentality is an **intra-**personal exercise of power and social control via a discourse. The use of discourses may get internalised by individuals which leads to more *efficient* forms of social control, as the discourse enables individuals to govern themselves by the *terms of that discourse ('the rules')*. To grossly simplify, a rule within Institutional Psychiatry's discourse is 'use pharmacological interventions for depression'. In the Moral Underclass discourse (outlined below) the rule for weight loss is 'eat less move more'.

If we accept this discourse, and internalise it, we will police ourselves by primarily attempting to change our individual behaviour and lifestyle choices. These methods are 'the rules'.

If a group can get their discourse accepted by everybody else as self-evidently true and correct, then there is no need for external policing to ensure the discourse is accepted. The recipient groups will do that. In this manner, policy makers and cultural commentators can broadcast their 'austerity' discourse of strivers v. skivers, hardworking families v. shirkers, deserving and undeserving poor and get the population to accept those narratives, and then there is less need to externally police behaviour through formal authority. Stigma will also do the job.

A *normative governmentality* is one in which we can become so immersed in a discourse that we become blind to it, as its world view is just 'obvious' to us. It is 'normal' and becomes part of our 'epistemic bubble' as it can exclude other ways of knowing. It becomes the lens through which we see the world.

Take for example the discourse of the 'war on drugs' based on 'prohibition'. It is *self-evident* (common sense) is it not, in this discourse, that cocaine and heroin are dangerous drugs and should be illegal, that they are highly addictive and kill people. It is *self-evident* that cannabis is a gateway drug to these 'harder drugs'. It is *self-evident* that we have to protect children from the 'pusher at the school gates'. It is *self-evident* that the only sane policy is prohibition, making it a criminal offence to purchase, use or distribute these drugs. If I believe this narrative to be self-evident and common sense, I will then self-police, by refraining from taking these drugs and will report anyone I know who does. This world view on drugs has of course been challenged as *not* self-evident and indeed is argued as mythological and counterproductive (Reinarman 2000; Cohen 2003).

If we turn this gaze towards everyday nursing practices, we might ask questions about the fundamental nature of the nurse–person interaction in various clinical fields. If Foucaldian perspectives are brought to bear to examine nurse communication, what might they possibly reveal?

Roberts (2005) uses just such a perspective to argue how power and knowledge are central to the process by which human beings are 'made subjects' and, therefore, how 'psychiatric identities' are produced. Roberts outlines explicit, everyday examples of the existence and exercise of power within psychiatry, such as compulsory admission and treatment of people under the Mental Health Act 1983. For example, the power of psychiatric categorisations and diagnoses are such that they can come to utterly overwhelm a person's identity. Roberts quotes R.D. Laing who suggested that within a psychiatric discourse: '*No one has schizophrenia, like having a cold. The patient has not got schizophrenia. He is schizophrenic*' (Roberts 2005, p. 34).

Roberts (2005) goes on to suggest that:

> a person is not thought to have schizophrenia while remaining 'essentially' the same; rather, schizophrenia is thought to 'split' or 'fragment' the very 'essence', the very being, of a person. To give a person a diagnosis of schizophrenia, therefore, is not to give a person one identity amongst others; instead, it is to suggest that a person is schizophrenic, that schizophrenia determines the very being of that person (p. 34).

The nurse and the person they work with can easily accept that identity and reinforce it in their language and relationships; if they do so they are exercising 'governmentality', policing themselves to conform to others' expectations, i.e. the expectations of traditional Institutional Psychiatry. It could be suggested that mental health nurses who uncritically operate within the culture of psychiatry and whose dominant mode of reflexivity is that of the communicative reflexive will be less likely to challenge the dominant discourse because for them consensus is most important.

In the next section, I further examine discourses that might be used to create a culture of professional practice in which the assumptions and values of the discourse becomes 'common sense' and 'taken for granted'. These discourses can be internalised and used to position the health professional as expert. They are also used to create a new self-identity as a professional. The agency of the nurse is again seen as an outcome of the interplay of structure, culture, their reflexive deliberations often in *taken for granted and common sense* contexts.

The biomedical discourse

It is arguable that biomedicine and its discourse dominates contemporary understandings of health and forms the basis of the NHS and other western health care systems (Jones 1994; Ion & Lauder 2015).

The biomedical model claims to be scientific. It sees itself as objective and reproducible, while the actual delivery of health care may be somewhat different. Many doctors incorporate other approaches, for example Narrative Medicine, Complementary and Alternative Medicine (CAMs) and a BioPsychoSocial approach.

The main tenets of biomedical discourse are:

1. Health is the 'absence of disease' and 'functional fitness'.
2. Health Services are geared mainly towards treating sick and disabled people.
3. A high value is put on the provision of specialist medical services, in mainly institutional settings, typically hospitals or clinics.
4. Doctors and other qualified experts diagnose illness and disease and sanction and supervise the withdrawal of service users from productive labour.
5. The main function of health services is remedial or curative – to get people back to productive labour.
6. Disease and sickness are explained within a biological framework that emphasises the physical nature of disease: that is, it is biologically reductionist.
7. Biomedicine works from a pathogenic origin of disease focus, emphasising risk factors and establishing abnormality (and normality).
8. Evidence-Based Practice: A high value is put on using scientific methods of research and on scientific knowledge. Qualitative evidence given by lay people or produced through academic research generally has a lower status as knowledge than quantitative evidence such as the Randomised Controlled Trial (RCT). (Source: adapted from Jones 1994)

Nurses might want to consider how an uncritical adoption of this discourse frames health and illness and delineates what can and cannot be done within a therapeutic relationship. It frames what is legitimate knowledge and can create a particular clinical culture. If this is the objective situation in which nurses' agency operates, we might want to think about how it then shapes nurses' 'concerns and projects' – what they think are priorities and appropriate courses of action. The same considerations can be applied to health inequalities.

Discourses on health inequalities

Carlisle (2001) outlines three discourses which seek to both explain health inequalities and to provide suggestions for courses of action on health inequalities. They are:

1.   The Redistribution discourse
2.   The Social Integrationist discourse
3.   The Moral Underclass discourse

Health professionals will be immersed and use these discourses perhaps unknowingly and uncritically. Any one of these discourses can provide the cultural landscape that explains human behaviour and outlines appropriate professional action.

An argument can be made that for many health professionals, particularly those not versed in public health theory and discourse, or in sociological theory on health inequalities, that the 'Moral Underclass discourse' provides for them the most salient explanation for health behaviour and outcomes. This discourse is part of the 'cultural thesis' that focuses on individual failure, poor moral choices, harmful cultural practices such as smoking, excess drinking, sedentary living, leading to ill health. The remedy within this discourse is education and information so that people should be empowered to make better cultural and lifestyle choices. The failure is individual, the remedy is individual based in education and lifestyle tips. In this discourse, the role of social structural issues such as the class/command dynamic (Scambler 2012) and socio-economic status in health inequalities, is either ignored, denied or unknown.

This discourse easily leads to 'lifestyle drift' (Hunter et al. 2009) responses to public health issues such as obesity as outlined in the following policy analysis.

The Foresight Report (Foresight 2007) on obesity identified the 'obesogenic environment' in which reductionist and mechanistic solutions, such as targeting obese individuals with messages about eating less and moving more, as only a small part of the solution. Foresight suggests there is no simple or single solution that works in a cause–effect way. 'Change 4 life' which focuses on individual **lifestyle changes** and **behaviour changes** will not be enough. This fails to engage with Foresight's 'whole systems approach'. Obesity has to be seen as a result of an interrelationship of factors (e.g. power relationships, poverty, employment). If responses are too narrow, focusing on individual lifestyle, the outcome will be failure and lifestyle drift.

Lifestyle Drift: This is the tendency for policy initiatives to recognise the need to take action on the wider determinants of health, e.g. as in the Foresight Report, but which as they get implemented they drift downstream to focus on individual lifestyle factors.

Lifestyle drift tends to move policy implementation away from measures that address social structural issues to measures that target the *most disadvantaged* groups in an attempt to deal with cultural issues such as smoking habits, food choices and exercise levels. As nurses work with individuals and families it is easy to see how lifestyle and behaviour change tools are attractive in their attempts to 'make every contact count'. Taking action on the wider determinants of health is more of a challenge for many clinically based nurses who work in secondary and primary care. This is because nurses often don't have either conceptual tools of analysis or control over social and economic factors such as housing.

Conclusion

A core concern of anthropology is that of culture but in a context. In this brief and partial exploration I have tried to suggest that there is a need to account for the interplay of social structure, culture and agency. I have suggested that the human self is not an autonomous self, free from society, making rational autonomous decisions. Rather the human self who acts does so within objective social and cultural contexts but not as a passive dupe of that context. The self is also a construct of society and culture but also constructs society and culture as culture flows through self and vice versa.

Inner conversations (reflexive deliberations) mediate the interplay of agency, structure and culture. If they did not and if we were cultural dopes, then nothing would change as the weight of custom, practice and tradition bear down upon us determining courses of action. Archer actually argues that autonomous reflexivity is becoming the more dominant mode rather than communicative reflexivity as tradition wanes in importance and guides to action are up for grabs. Foucault's work asks us to consider how discourses can frame reality and thus provide an aspect of that context in which the human agent acts. Taken for granted, common sense, uncritical and unreflexive practice merely perpetuate systems of health care that *in extremis* can be oppressive and dehumanising.

For health inequalities and public health interventions there does seem to be a tension between explanations using individualist discourses focusing on the unhealthy cultural practices of an 'underclass' and other explanations that understand wider determinants of health that transcends individual decision making. All of this means the study of structure, agency and culture provides interesting lines of enquiry for nurses.

References

Alvesson M & Skoldberg K (2000) Reflexive Methodology – New Vistas for Qualitative research, Sage, London.

American Anthropological Association (2017) *What is Anthropology?* (http://www.americananthro.org, accessed 28 November 2017).

Archer M S (1982) Morphogenesis versus structuration: On combining structure and action, *British Journal of Sociology*, 33(4), 455–483.

Archer M S (1988) *Culture and Agency: The Place of Culture in Social Theory*, Cambridge University Press, Cambridge.

Archer M S (1995) *Realist Social Theory: The Morphogenetic Approach*, Cambridge University Press, Cambridge.

Archer M S (2000) *Being Human: The Problem of Agency*, Cambridge University Press, Cambridge.

Archer M S (2003) *Structure, Agency and the Internal Conversation*, Cambridge University Press, Cambridge.

Archer M S (2007) *Making our Way through the World: Human Reflexivity and Social Mobility*, Cambridge University Press, Cambridge.

Archer M S (2008) *Culture and Agency: The Place of Culture in Social Theory*, 2nd Edition, Cambridge University Press, Cambridge.

Archer M S (2010) *Reflexivity*, (https://www.scribd.com/document/142679395/Reflexivity, accessed 28 February 2018).

Archer M S (2012) *The Reflexive Imperative in Late Modernity*, Cambridge University Press, Cambridge.

Carlisle S (2001) Inequalities in health: Contested explanations, shifting discourses and ambiguous policies, *Critical Public Health*, 11(3), 267–281.

Cohen P (2003) The drug prohibition church and the adventure of reformation, *International Journal of Drug Policy*, 14(2), 213–215.

Davies B and HarreR (1990) *Positioning: The discursive production of selves*, *Journal for the Theory of Social Behaviour*, 20, 43–63.

Engelke M (2017a) *How to Think Like an Anthropologist*, Pelican, London.

Engelke M (2017b) *How to Think like an Anthropologist*, RSA Events, 2 November (https://soundcloud.com/the_rsa/how-to-think-like-an-anthropologist, accessed 28 November 2017).

Foresight (2007) *Tackling Obesities: Future Choices* (https://www.gov.uk/government/uploads/system/uploads/attachment_data/file/287937/07-1184x-tackling-obesities-future-choices-report.pdf, accessed 28 February 2018).

Foucault M (1963) *The Birth of the Clinic: An Archaeology of Medical Perception*, Routledge, London.

Foucault M (1969) *The Archaeology of Knowledge and the Discourse on Language*, translated from the French by A M Sheridan Smith, Pantheon Books, New York.

Foucault M (1975) *Discipline and Punish: The Birth of the Prison*, Routledge, London.

Garfinkel H (1974) The origins of the term ethnomethodology. In R Turner (Ed.), *Ethnomethodology*, 15–18, Penguin, Harmondsworth.

Grant A (2015) Demedicalising misery: Welcoming the human paradigm in mental health nurse education, *Nurse Education Today*, 35(9), e50–53.

Grant A & Goodman B (2018) *Communication and Interpersonal Skills for Nurses*, 4th Edition, Esp. Chapter 11, Sage, London.

Ion R and Lauder W (2015) Willis and the generic turn in nursing, *Nurse Education Today*, 35(7), 841–842.

Hunter D J, Popay J, Tannahill C, Whitehead M & Elson T (2009) *Marmot Review Working Committee 3. Cross-cutting sub-group report: Learning Lessons from the Past: Shaping a Different Future*, Institute of Health Equity, London.

Jones L (1994) *The Social Context of Health and Health Care*, Macmillan, Basingstoke.

Lakoff G (2004) *Don't think of an Elephant: Know your Values and Frame the Debate*, Chelsea Green, Vermont.

Minnich E (2017) *The Evil of Banality: The Life and Death Importance of Thinking*, Rowman and Littlefield, Lanham.

Moore J (2018) *I'm Depressed about Antidepressants* (https://fiddaman.blogspot.co.uk/2018/02/guest-post-im-depressed-about.html?m=1#.WpgBx2acZUf, accessed 1 March 2018).

Orwell G (1941) *England your England: Part 1 of the Lion and the Unicorn*, Penguin, London.

Reinarman C (2000) The Dutch example shows that liberal drug laws can be beneficial. In S Barbour (ed.), *Drug Legalization: Current Controversies*, 102–108, Greenhaven Press, San Diego.

Roberts M (2005) The production of the psychiatric subject: Power, knowledge and Michel Foucault, *Nursing Philosophy*, 6(1), 33–42.

Royal Anthropological Institute (2017) *What is Anthropology?* (https://www.discoveranthropology.org.uk/about-anthropology/what-is-anthropology.html, accessed 28 November 2017).

Scambler G (2012) *GBH: Greedy Bastards and Health Inequalities* (http://www.grahamscambler.com/gbh-greedy-bastards-and-health-inequalities/, accessed 28 February 2018).

Scambler G (2013a) *Archer and the Focused Autonomous Reflexive* (http://www.grahamscambler.com/archer-and-the-focused-autonomous-reflexive/, accessed 28 February 2018).

Scambler G (2013b) *Archer and the Dedicated Meta Reflexive* (http://www.grahamscambler.com/archer-and-the-dedicated-meta-reflexive/, accessed 28 February 2018).

Scambler G (2013c) *Archer and the Vulnerable Fractured Reflexive* (http://www.grahamscambler.com/archer-and-the-vulnerable-fractured-reflexive/, accessed 28 February 2018).

Scambler G (2013d) Resistance in unjust times: Archer, structured agency and the sociology of health inequalities, *Sociology*, 47(1), 142–156.

Smith S & Grant A (2016) The corporate construction of psychosis and the rise of psychosocial paradigm: Emerging implications for mental health nursing education, *Nurse Education Today*, 39, 22–25.

Sundin-Huard D (2001) Subject positions theory – its application to understanding collaboration (and confrontation) in critical care, *Journal of Advanced Nursing*, 34(3), 376–382.

Further reading

1 Alvesson M & Skoldberg K (2000) *Reflexive Methodology – New Vistas for Qualitative Research*, Sage, London.
2 Aronowitz R, Deener A, Keene D, Schnittker J & Tach L (2015) Cultural reflexivity in health research and practice, *American Journal of Public Health*, 2015 July, 105 (Suppl 3).
3 Etherington K (2004) *Becoming a Reflexive Researcher: Using Our Selves in Research*, Jessica Kingsley, London.

INDEX

Aamodt, A. A. 41
Abel-Smith, B. 26, 90
Adams, V. 95
Allan, H. 30
Allen, D. 27
Alvesson, M. 149
American Civil War 103
anthropologist; *see also* cultural anthropology
anthropology: culture and 2–7; definition of 146;
    early development of 4; literature on nursing
    and 7–10; method of 8; for nursing 1, 11, 13;
    of nursing 1, 12, 13, 14, 15; principles of 1;
    subfields of 1, 15, 146; *see also* medical
    anthropology and nursing anthropology
Antonacopoulou, E. P. 59
apprenticeship: in clinical environment 85, 87–8,
    health care workforce 87; learning by doing,
    and learning by being with an expert 87–8
Archer, M. 147, 148, 149, 150, 159
Archer, Margaret 145
Arendt, H. 101
Aries, P. 136
armchair anthropologist 4–5, 36, 39
Ashforth, B. E. 123
Ashley, J. A. 26
Asylums (Goffman) 23, 47
Atkinson, P. 37, 39
Auger, J. A. 136
Australian Aborigines 3–4
Australian health care 4, 5
autonomous reflexivity 150, 151, 159

Bangladesh: nursing work in 109
Bates, C. 71
bathing 77–8, 120, 123, 125
Beals, R. L. 29

Bell, C. 70
Benedict, R. 5, 6
Bharj, K. 118
biomedical discourse 152–3, 157, 159
blood: cultural perceptions of 118; in health care,
    importance of 118; -related rituals 117–18
Boas, F. 6
body ideal 121–2
body(ies): anthropological view of 114, 115,
    116–17; definition of 114; individual 116; in
    nursing work 113, 114–16, 120–5; M. Douglas
    115; physical 115, 116; social 115, 116; theory
    of 'two' 115, 116; uniqueness of human 121;
    Scheper-Hughes & Lock's theory of three 116
body image 121–2
body politic 116–17, 118
body presentation 121, 122
body reality 121
Brink, P. J. 11, 12, 42
Brooks, I. 62
Brown, R. B. 62
Bruni, N. 9
Bryan, L. 132
Bueno, C. F. 1
Bullough, B. 2
Bullough, V. L. 2
Burgess, R. G. 39

Callahan, D. 131
Caplan, P. 117
capping ceremony 71
Carlisle, S. 158
Carpenter, D. R. 37, 39, 108
Chapman, C. 73, 74
Chief Nursing Officer's 6Cs 154–5
Chrisman, N. J. 11

Cirlot, J. E. 137
Clifford, J. 36
Coming of Age in Samoa (Mead) 6, 39
common sense 146–7, 159
communal resocialisation agencies
    85, 86–7
communicative reflexivity 150, 159
Costello, J. 132
Crimean War: nursing during 3, 107, 115
critical care unit (CCU): characteristics of 130;
    cultural scene 30–30; end-of-life care in
    129–30, 137; life-sustaining technology in 130,
    133–4; nurses and
    patient family relations in 135–6; patient
    privacy in 136
cultural anthropology 1, 2, 12
culture shock 84
cultural transference 83
culture: definitions of 2, 5–7, 28, 38–9, 146, 148;
    as dynamic process 9, 10; functionalist view of
    6; human agency and 145–6, 147; importance
    of 146; in nursing work 10, 20 145; scholarly
    debates on meaning of 6, 20; social structure
    and 145–6, 148; *see also* culture shock
Cypress, B. S. 132

D'Antonio, P. 103
Davidhizar, R. E. 56
Davies, B. 151, 152
Davies, C. 27
death: concept of good 132, 133; as disturbance
    of social order 129, 132, 134, 135; as failure
    137–8; notion of 'bad' 135; social 136–7; as
    treated disease, perception of 131
death and dying: in critical care unit, study of 129;
    cultural environment of 129, 141–2; creating a
    space for 131; family members' dealing with
    140–1; life support technology and 133–4;
    liminality of 129, 134–5; nurses' perception of
    61–2, 130, 132–3, 135–6, 137–8; patient
    awareness of 132; social aspect of 132–4,
    136–7; spatial aspect of 61, 129, 131–2,
    135–6; symbolism of bedside curtains 129, 132,
    133, 139; temporality of 135–6; in Western
    society, perception of 133, 134, 136, 137;
    see also withdrawal of treatment
De Craemer, W. 77, 78
De Santis, L. 11, 14
Dickens, C. 105
Dick, P. 120
dirt and pollution: anthropological observations of
    114–15, 119; in hospitals 119; as 'matter out of
    place' 119; notion of order in relation to 119;
    in nursing work 113–14, 120–5; in relation to
    the body 113, 120, 124; social and moral
    aspects of 119–20, 123–4
dirty work 123, 125

discourse: concept of 152–3; biomedical 157; on
    health inequalities 158
discursive practices in nursing culture 151–2
disease 124
Dobson, S. 11
Dorcy, K. S. 23, 59
Dougherty, M. 11, 13
Douglas, M. 77, 115, 116, 118–19,
    120, 123, 124
Duchscher, J. E. B. 85

Eastern Hospitals and English Nurses (Taylor) 3,
    115–16
Easthope, G. 85, 86, 87
Edgecombe, N. 42
Engebretson, J. 11
Engelke, M. 146
Enrolled Nurse *see* registered nurse
ethnographic fieldwork 4, 36, 37, 38, 39, 44,
    45, 138
ethnographic research 40, 47–8
ethnographies of nursing: published doctoral
    studies on 45–7; unpublished doctoral
    studies on 43–5
ethnography: anthropological lens 47;
    characteristics of 37–8; development of 38–41;
    insider's and outsider's views of 43; as
    methodology 37, 38; myths about 41–2; as
    narrative 36; in nursing research 37, 41–3; and
    promotion of colonial policy 39
ethnomethodology 146
European Nursing Directive 93
euthanasia 131
Evans-Pritchard, E. E. 39
Ewan, C. E. 32, 84

Fealy, G. 86
Fenwick, E. B. 2, 24, 26,
    89–90, 110
Florence Nightingale Foundation 107
Ford, P. 72, 73
Foucault, Michel 145, 146, 153, 155
fractured reflexivity 150
framing in nursing culture 151
Frankenberg, R. 40, 41
Fry, E. 2

Gamarnikow, E. 116
Geertz, C. 4, 36
Geissler, W. 2, 15
Gerry, C. J. 104
Giger, J. N. 56
Giroux, H. A. 46
Glaser, B. G. 69, 74, 133, 136
Gluckman, M. 40
Goffman, E. 23–4, 47
Goodale, J. 118

Gordon, S. 26
Gourley, J. 4, 5
governmentality 155, 156
Grant, S. 104
Grey, Peter 51
Grint, K. 53, 101, 102

Hadley, M. B. 109
Hagey, R. 3, 5
Halford, S. 63
Hallam, E. 135
Hall, E. T. 56, 63
handover report: ritual, 94
Harre, R. 151, 152
health care: in Australia 4, 5; changes in 82;
    importance of blood in 118; in Russia 104;
    in the United States 58
Hector, Winifred 25, 26
Helman, Cecil 7, 28, 56, 69, 74
Henderson, Virginia 33, 52, 99
Hendry, J. 119
Hockey, J. 61, 135
Hodder, I. 5
Holden, P. 11, 12, 13, 29, 107
Holland, K. 40, 75, 133, 135, 147
hospice 55, 61
hospital: association with dirt 119; authority
    distribution in 31; as cornerstone of health care
    system 81; economic system within 31–2;
    moral purpose of 55–6; organisational culture
    of 31; time and space in 55–6, 135–6;
    timetables in 58; as workplace 55; ward design
    of 60; *see also* surgical wards
hospital set 86–7; *see also* Set, the
Huch, R. K. 4
Hughes, E. 123
human agency: culture and 145–6, 147, 148;
    definition of 147, 148; modes of operation of
    149; and the 'self' 147; social structure and
    145–6, 147, 148
Hunt, S. 43
hygiene 119
hypertension 153–4

Illich, I. 133
illness: *vs.* disease and sickness 124–5; as identity
    156; social impact of 53–4
India: development of nursing in 5, 27, 108; status
    of nurses in 25, 27, 109; veneration of Florence
    Nightingale in 109, 110
Infante, M. S. 85, 87
initiation of student nurses: cultural context and
    90, 94–6; link between ritual and 69, 70;
    placement as context for 91–3; spatial context
    of **91**, 93–4; structure and organisation of 94;
    temporal context of 90, 93; tribal roots of 82
inner conversations 147, 149, 150, 159

intensive care 138
Intensive Care Society (ICS) 131
intensive care units (ICU) 43, 45, 74, 129, 131,
    133–4, 136
intensive therapy units (ITU) 73, 122
intuition in nursing 73

Jacka, K. 87
Japan: culture studies 5; daily hygiene in 119;
    development of nursing, 106; HIV/Hepatitis C
    patient care in 118; veneration of Florence
    Nightingale in 106
Japanese Red Cross Society 106
Jervis, L. L. 125
Johnson, S. E. 109, 110
Johnson, S. J. 45
Jones, A. 56, 63
Jones, T. L. 63–4
Jowsey, T. 60

Kaiserworth: daily routines at 51, 57, 64
Kalisch, B. J. 83, 105
Kalisch, P. A. 83, 105
Kaminski, J. 21
Katz, P. 122
Kirchhoff, K. T. 133
Kleinman, A. 124, 125
knowledge and power 153, 154
knowledgeable doer 89
Kramer, M. 84
Kreiner, G. E. 123
Kuper, A. 38, 39

labour: *vs.* work 101
La Fontaine, J. S. 68, 69, 72, 75,
    90, 91, 117
Laing, R. D. 156
Lakoff, G. 151
language of medicine 153
Lavenda, R. H. 1
Lawler, J. 61, 122
Lawton, D. 23
learning to be a nurse: becoming a
    registered nurse 89; dual role reality 84;
    the Set 86–87; two parallel settings
    or segments 84
Leininger, M. 7, 9, 10, 11, 12
Leininger's Sunrise Model 9
Leonard, P. 63
Lewin, D. 87
liberal human self 148
lifestyle drift responses 145, 158
liminality 134
Littlewood, J. 11–13, 28–9, 53, 55, 60,
    107, 120, 125
Lock, M. 116, 118, 121
Loudan, J. B. 70

Macdonald, S. 62
MacGuire, G. 22–3, 70, 86
Mahoney, J. S. 11
Malinowski, B. 6, 36, 39, 45
Mallidou, A. A. 26
man of modernity 147
Manthey, M. 58
Marcus, G. F. 36
Maric, T. 72
Martinez, L. 119
McClaren, P. L. 46
McKenna, M. 11
McLaren, P. 83, 89
Mead, M. 6, 22, 33, 39, 87
medical anthropology 2, 13, 15–16
medical doctors: deskilling of 102
Melia, K. 47, 62, 75, 81, 84, 93
Melosh, B. 24
menstruation 117, 118
Mental Health Act (1983) 156
mentors: as gatekeepers 95
Menzies, I. E. P. 73, 76
Merton, R. 76
meta reflexivity 150
midwives 118
Miller, A. 134
Minnich, E. 149
Moral Underclass discourse 155–6, 158
Mulhall, A. 11, 13, 14, 15

Nair, S. 109
named nurse 58, 59
National Health Service (NHS) 58, 103, 151, 157
negotiated space 27
Nightingale, Florence: as armchair anthropologist
    4–5, 36; correspondence of 5; on design of
    surgical wards 60; on importance of cleanliness
    125; international reputation of 27, 106–7,
    110; legacy of 2, 5, 21, 23, 84, 105–6; model
    of nursing of 105–6; rituals in honour of 70,
    71, 107; as symbol of nursing profession 84,
    109–10; view of nursing training 24; visit to
    Kaiserworth 57; writings of 3, 4, 5
Nightingale School of Nursing 21, 107
Nightingale wards 23, 63, 94
Noble, M. 7, 8
normative governmentality 156
nurse-doctor interactions 27, 30, 132, 152
nurse-patient encounters 14–15, 31, 132, 135,
    137, 152–3
nurses: bathing of patients by 123; changing role
    of 82–3; contribution to hygiene 116; as
    cultural group 12, 28–9; daily routine of
    27–8, 51, 57, 64; dead bodies and 124;
    decision-making process 58; definitions of 33;
    dirty work of 125; doctors' relations with 27,
    30, 132; male 124; night shifts 62; patient'

relations with 14–15, 31, 132, 135, 137,
    152–3; patient's family and 129, 131, 132, 135;
    perception of death by 132; popular image of
    33, 105–6; professional socialisation of 32–3;
    registration of 26, 75; social status of 25, 27,
    108; subject positioning of 151–2; uniform of
    71; work time of 31–2
Nurses Registration Act (1919) 26
nurse training: apprenticeship system 24–5;
    curriculum 23; debates about 25; duration of
    25; history of 21–2, 26–7; hospital
    environment and 24; Labour Party policy for
    26; medical model of 24–5; men in nursing
    124; Nightingale's model for 23–4; set system
    approach 22; student hierarchy 22–3
nursing: American Civil War and 103;
    anthropology and 7–15; vs. biomedicine 13;
    as body work 120–3; in Canadian stroke unit
    62–3; changes to 104; 'code burgundy' issue
    and 63; concept of sick 103; during Crimean
    War 3, 107, 115; critical care 134; cultural
    transference in 83–4; as culture 20, 28–31, 33;
    definitions of 52–3, 78, 99; deskilling in 102–3;
    development of modern 21–6, 27; as dirty
    work 123–6; ethnographic research of 29; first
    training school of 21–2; as form of emotional
    labour 101, 102; vs. medicine 13; as occupation
    21, 25; in Japan 106; origin of 21; popular
    perception of 104–5; as profession 2–3, 10, 11,
    21; reciprocity in 95–6; regulations of 26;
    scholarly literature on 11; in a submarine 63; in
    Russia 104; temporal landscape of night 62; as
    women's domestic labour 33, 108
Nursing and Midwifery Council (NMC) 53, 70,
    75, 101, 103
nursing anthropology 11, 12, 16, 25, 46
nursing culture: authority in 31;
    communication system 32; discursive
    practices of 151–2; economic system of 31–2;
    framing in 151; human agency and 149;
    language in 153, 156–7; modes of reflexivity
    151, 152, 155; social structures in 31, 32;
    studies of 44–6; transition as part of 81–2;
    types of 14–15
nursing-medical boundary negotiations 27
nursing rituals: of bathing 77–8, 120; capping
    ceremony 71–2; criticism of 72–3; daily
    routine and 76–7; of the handover report 32,
    62, 77, 94, 95; in the operating room 122; as
    part of nursing culture 78; related to
    admission and discharge of patient from
    hospital 77; related to death and dying 74, 77;
    studies of 73–4, 76–7; symbolism and 44–5;
    system of 29, 30; therapeutic 77;
    types of 73; see also initiation of nurses; rituals
nursing space 62, 63
nursing time 62, 64

nursing work: body in 114–15, 126; changes to 102–3; conditions of 53, 99, 100–1, 126; in different cultural contexts 107–10, 111; dirt and pollution associated with 108–9, 113; meaning of 52–3, 102; in political context 102; spatial contexts of 51, 59; student nursing work 53; temporal context of 51, 57; in the US 103

Oakley, A. 108
obesity 145, 146–7, 148–9, 158; obesogenic environment 149, 158

Ohnuki-Tierney, E. 119
Olsen, V. L. 86
Orwell, G. 148
Osborne, O. H. 8

Papadopoulos, I. 10
Parsons, T. 29, 30
patients: relations with nurses 14–15, 31, 132, 135, 137, 152–3; spatial experience of 60; student nurses and 95–6; subject positioning of 151
Pattison, N. 133, 134
Philpin, S. 44–5, 62, 73, 77, 83, 122, 134
Picco, E. 121
placements: bounded placements 91; context of initiation 91; time and space in 53; see also student nurses
Pool, R. 2, 15
pollution 77, 113
positioning: concept of 151, 152
Pountney, L. 72
Price, B. 121
Primary Nursing 58–9
Project 2000 26, 89; see also knowledgeable doer 89
psychiatry 156–7
purification: removal of dirt 77

Radcliffe-Brown, A. R. 6
Rafferty, A. M. 21, 25, 108, 110
Ramsden, I. M. 10
Realist tale 54
Redistribution discourse 158
reflexivity mode 148, 149–50, 151, 152
registered nurse 75, 83, 89–90, 100, 101
Representation of the People Act (1918) 24
Reverby, S. M. 108, 118
Richman, J. 41
rites of passage 69, 75, 85, 107, 134; key stages in 68–78; incorporation 69, 75, 83; separation 83; transition 81–85
ritual: definitions of 68–9, 72, 77; functions of 69; initiation and 69–72; public and private elements of 70; purpose of 69; religions and 70; ritualism 76; routine and 72–4; scholarly literature on 68–72; 'schooling' as performance

of 83; social status and 69, 75; symbols and 70, 73, 74–5; see also nursing rituals
ritualism, definition of in nursing 76
Roberts, M. 156
Roques, A. 109
Rosen, G. 81
Roth, J. 47, 57

St Bart's Hospital 25
St Thomas's Hospital 21–2, 84
Salih, S. 84
Salisbury, R. F. 8
Savage, J. 42, 60, 61
Scambler, G. 147, 150
Scheper-Hughes, N. 116, 118, 121
Schmalenberg, C. 84
schooling 85, 88–9
schools of nursing 21–2
Schultz, E. A. 1, 69
Seacole, M. 84, 105, 110
Seale, C. 132, 133
Seaton, L. P. 10, 14
Seccombe, I. 101
Selanders, L. C. 105, 106
self 147, 153; see also liberal human self
Selimiye Barracks 107
Seneviratne, C. C. 62, 63
Sera-Shriar, E. 4
Seymour, J. 83, 130, 133, 134
Sharp, R. 95
Shebini, N. 58
Sheiman, I. 104
Shepherd, S. M. 10
sickness 53–5, 125
Silberger, M. R. 73, 78
Simpson, A. 113, 119, 123
Simpson, R. 113, 119, 123, 124
Skoldberg, K. 149
Slevin, O. 89
Smith, P. 102
social anthropology 8–9, 12
social integrationist discourse 158
social interactionism 6
socialisation 83, 85
social structures 147–8
'social system' theory 29–30
Somjee, G. 108
space: bounded 60; definition of 59; cultural 130; dimensions of 60; for dying 131; in life of nurses 51; movement in 63; negotiated space 27; public and private 55; relationship between learning and 59–60; of sick people 54–5, 61; symbolic 60
Spradley, J. P. 41, 42
status passage 69; see also rites of passage
Stocking, G. W. 5
Strauss, A. 55, 69, 74, 133, 136

Street, A. 46, 47
Streubert, H. J. 37, 39
student nurses (probationers): apprenticeship of
    87–8; bounded placements experiences for **91**,
    91–2; clinical experience of 89; communal
    resocialisation of 86–7; dual reality of 84–5, 88;
    education and training of 26, 88–9, 93, 94–5;
    fields of practice 92; 'hidden curriculum' of 94;
    initiation of 90–6; patients' relations with 95–6;
    learning to become a nurse 81; knowledgeable
    doer 89; placements 53, 60, 61, 81–2;
    professional Code of Conduct 92–3;
    socialisation of 85; 'stripping away of self'
    process 86; time and space of 51, 89–90;
    transitions of 85, 94; vulnerability of 95
Sudnow, D. 136
Sundin-Huard, D. 152
Suominen, T. 29
surgical wards 60–1; *see also* hospital wards;
    see also symbolic space
Svensson, R. 27
Symonds, A. 43
Synnott, A. 114, 115

Takahashi, A. 106
Taylor, F. M. 3
Templeman, J. 74
time: cultural dimension of 56–7; monochronic
    56; of nursing work 51, 53; polychronic 56; of
    sick person 54–5; social and clock 31–2, 57; of
    surgery 57–8; temporality 135; with and
    without space 63; Zerubavel 31, 55, 57
timetables in health care delivery 57–8
total patient care 8
transcultural nursing (TCN) 7, 9, 10–11, 14, 56
transition: liminality 75; three key stages 75; shock
    85; *see also* rites of passage
transition to becoming a nurse 81–2, 83, 85
tribal societies: blood-related rituals in 117–18;
    ethnographic studies of 99–100; transitions in 83
Tripp-Reimer, T. 11, 13
Turner, V. 32, 45, 46, 69–70, 74, 77, 83, 135
Twigg, J. 60, 120, 125

Tylor, E. B. 2, 5, 7, 38–9

United States: Equal Franchise Act (1928) 24;
    health care in 58; nurses training in 26–7;
    nursing work in 103

Van Gennep, A. 45–6, 69–70, 75, 77, 81,
    83, 85, 134
Van Maanen, J. 3, 40, 47, 54
Victorian Health Reform 4
Vogel, E. F. 5
Voget, F. W. 5, 6
Vouzavali, F. J. D. 132

Wada, K. 118
Wakefield, A. 63
Walker, V. H. 73, 76, 77
Walsh, M. J. 72, 73
Walter, T. 136
ward design 60–61, 64, 93–94
Wheeler, S. 85
White, R. 32, 84
Whittaker, E. W. 86
Wicks, D. 27
Wilkins, H. 9
Williams, A. 43
withdrawal of treatment: bedside curtains
    and 139, 141; death of patient after 140–1;
    decision-making process of 129, 131,
    138, 139; management of 132, 138–41;
    moral considerations of 133–4; nurses' role in
    140–1; patient's family and 138, 140;
    preparations for 138, 139–40;
    UK guidelines for 131
Wolf, Z. R. 45, 61, 73, 77–8, 120, 125
women: association with pollution 118;
    emancipation of 2, 24; nursing and 33, 108
work: definition of 101, 102; *vs.* labour 101; *see
    also* nursing work

Young, A. 124

Zerubavel, E. 31, 55, 57–8, 61, 62, 93

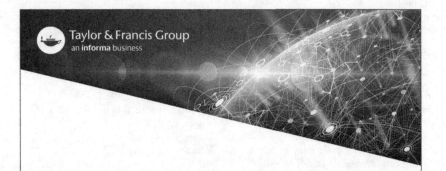

Printed in the United States
by Baker & Taylor Publisher Services